HEALING STORIES THAT WILL CHANGE YOUR LIFE

Linda,

You are the

Best

♡

D Katok

HEALING STORIES THAT WILL CHANGE YOUR LIFE

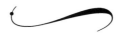

Dr. Kate Keville

ISBN-13: 9781546953258
ISBN-10: 1546953256
Library of Congress Control Number: 2017908753
CreateSpace Independent Publishing Platform
North Charleston, South Carolina

DEDICATION

This book is dedicated to Alice and Chris Dorrance whose generous gifts and continued support of the Mesa Refuge Writers Residency program have been instrumental in the creation of the pages that you are about to read.

I would also like to thank every loving person who has crossed my threshold over the last two decades seeking answers. Without you and your treasured trust the solutions and options explored within these pages would likely remain unknown.

NATIVE QUECHUA FABLE

A FIRE RAGED in the forest. As the blaze continued one-by-one all of the animals of the forest fled. In the middle of the chaos, a lone hummingbird flew to a nearby river, dove into the water, and filled its tiny beak. The hummingbird then swooped over the fire and dropped the water from its beak hoping to quell the raging flames below. The hummingbird continued back and forth for hours and hours.

A deer, puzzled by the bird's efforts, asked "Why don't you run away with us hummingbird? You will never be able to put that fire out. Even a million of your tiny trips will never be enough." The hummingbird replied, "That may be true wise deer. Perhaps I could fly for all of eternity and spit an ocean of drips and the fire would still rage on. Yet, I will continue to do what I must in order to do my part. Doing my part makes my hummingbird heart hum."

This Quechua Fable to me shows the analogy of the trillion dollar pharmaceutical industry, which is the forest fire, and the Holistic Health industry being the Hummingbird. Our traditional healthcare is in a crisis, treating chronic health issues with crisis care methods. Even though the initial results may be quick, long term usage of pharmaceuticals cause many irreversible side effects. Holistic Healthcare, may take longer, as the body takes time to heal from chronic health problems, such as the small hummingbird tries to put out the fire, but in the end, one's quality of life will be better.

Like the hummingbird in the story above, I am compelled to "do my part." I hope this book enables practitioners and non-practitioners alike to see that every health issue is multi-faceted.

Particularly in the Western Hemisphere, we tend to seek out and exclusively rely upon a doctor's diagnosis, treatment, and drug remedy. The media has recently shined a light on the devastating effects of prescription drug addiction. Hundreds of thousands of patients have ended up with dangerous and even deadly side-effects and consequences simply as a result of following the doctor's orders.

On a positive note, this recent epidemic has inspired people all over the globe to dig a little deeper and find answers for themselves. To seek out more natural, holistic methods and treatments rather than to play another risky game of roulette with commonly prescribed synthetic drugs with potentially hazardous side effects.

With nearly twenty-five years of experience I am happy to report great success employing and adapting some of these alternative treatments, from utilizing Neurofeedback and Craniosacral Therapy to Neurological Integration System, and Holographic Health. These techniques have been varied but the outcomes have all been similar.

I have witnessed hundreds of success stories and am so excited to share some of these accounts with you. This book contains some of the most memorable, remarkable, and poignant stories of patients who, as Robert Frost described in his famous poem, "took the one (road) less traveled." Patients who traded traditional treatments for less orthodox methods and as a result of that choice now live happier and healthier lives today.

INTRODUCTION

THE HUMAN BODY has enchanted me ever since I can remember. As a child I was on a treasure hunt to discover the cause of my breathing difficulties. Prepared for my near daily attacks, an inhaler remained stashed in my lunchbox throughout my school years. My Irish grandmother first introduced me to the healing power of plants when I was 19. That lit a spark inside me and fanned my curiosity toward more holistic healing methods. For the last three decades I've studied everything from anatomy and physiology, reflexology, iridology to biomechanics and nutrition. I received a doctorate of Chiropractic Healthcare and have provided Chiropractic care for two of those three decades. The healing masters I have had the opportunity to study with are among the most revered on the planet. I am truly blessed for every lesson they've imparted.

My goal has been to teach my patients and loved ones the premise that the human body is an amazing self-healing miracle. When we understand that in a state of balance, our bodies will heal itself, we will live a life of high energy, love, and peace. It is my observation, when the body is in a state of imbalance, or dis-ease, we are sick.

With a spirit of love, universal intention and the hope for a betterment of mankind I feel obliged to pass along these lessons which have indelibly informed my years of healing experience.

My goal with each patient has always been to remain truthful and helpful. As a result of that commitment certain truths have

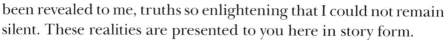
been revealed to me, truths so enlightening that I could not remain silent. These realities are presented to you here in story form.

My ultimate desire is that you benefit from these stories. That you read this book and consequently feel inspired to think deeply and independently and to consider options outside of the constraints of Western medicine.

Bear in mind that the healthcare and pharmaceutical industries are not necessarily looking out for the health and wellness of Americans. These mega-trillion dollar industries are money-making machines. With our political system in lock step with these giants we are rarely privy to the whole picture. Secrecy has been very profitable for some. These industries would prefer that you remain in the disempowered dark and tethered to the mercy of their expensive medications. Unfortunately, patients like you and me pay the ultimate price in more ways than one.

I intend no harm. I swore that oath with my hand planted squarely on my heart the day I received my doctorate. My aim is not to defame or discredit the hard work of other health professionals, many of whom are dedicated and caring. My only objective is to present you with "my side of the story" so that you, the healthcare consumer, can begin to make more informed conscious decisions regarding your healthcare.

The following stories are intentionally presented in no particular order enabling the reader to pick up the book, thumb quickly through, and randomly select any story on any page without effort.

Excluding family members, names have been changed to protect patient confidentiality. All the stories presented here have been derived from contemporaneous practice notes.

If you find value in these stories, I invite you to spread the word. Perhaps together we can change the hearts and minds of those seeking enlightenment regarding their health, happiness, and well-being.

Love and healing,
Dr. Kate Keville

TABLE OF CONTENTS

Dedication v
Native Quechua Fable vii
Introduction ix

Karen: Anxiety, Indigestion, Insomnia 1
Logan: Car Accident Injuries 3
Ralph: Complications From a Previous Accident 5
Nathan: Strep 7
Kimberly: Raynaud's Syndrome and Scleroderma 8
Amber: Chronic Neck, Back and Shoulder Pain 12
Anthony: Chronic Asthma 13
Freeda: Fibromyalgia 15
John: Stomach Problems 17
Robin: Allergies 18
Jimmy: Chemotherapy Side Effects 20
Tara: Carpal Tunnel, Allergies 23
Conor: Schizophrenia 25
Joshua: Graves' Disease 27
Margaret: Severe Back Pain 29
Gary: Chronic Fatigue, Depression 31
Michael: Autism 36
Randy: Low Back Pain 39
Katlyn: Seizures 40
Sarah: Lupus 41
Ann: Tingling Electrical Shocks 44
Bill: Heavy Metal Poisoning 45

Bobbie: Chronic Shoulder Pain 47
Brenda: Gallbladder Congestion. 48
Katherine: Chronic Neck Pain 50
Cecil: Chronic Back Pain, Depression 52
Dennis: Chronic Skin Problems 54
Maria: Grand Mal Seizures 56
Pat: Chronic Hip Pain 58
Theresa: Partial Paralyzation 59
Betsy: Chronic Elbow Pain 61
Melissa: Urinary Tract Infections 63
Katie: Postpartum Depression. 65
Jack: Hip And Knee Pain. 67
Gaffney: Depression, Anger 68
Kevil: Testicular Cancer. 70
Dr Kate: Asthma. 73

Conclusion · 77
The Benefits of Echo Hydrogen Enriched Water 79
Alternative Techniques and Systems. 85
About the Author. 91

KAREN: ANXIETY, INDIGESTION, INSOMNIA

KAREN SOUGHT MY help over 13 years ago. She suffered ongoing anxiety, indigestion, insomnia, and a rapid heartbeat. Every time she visited her primary care physician she was sent home with a different drug. Each drug seemed to exacerbate her symptoms. Her acid reflux medication seemed to create even more digestive distress and her psychotropic medications only caused her anxiety to spike.

Karen's angst and unease was especially perplexing. She explained "I have nothing to be worried over. I have a beautiful family, an amazing business, yet I suffer daily." Karen was loved, revered, and cherished by her family and friends. She was also profiled in Forbes magazine for her business acumen and achievements.

Surprisingly, my testing revealed an incident of food poisoning in Karen's past. Karen confirmed that she did indeed suffer a serious bout of food poisoning when travelling through Mexico several years prior.

She was puzzled. "How could a short spell of food poisoning from years ago continue to upset my system?" she wondered. I explained how salmonella, along with many other food poisons, can remain deep in intestinal tissues for years. Our 33-foot long stretch of intestines provides plenty of places for bacteria-secreting poisons to find a home.

This poison is discharged 24-hours a day, causing inflammation of the intestines, stomach, gallbladder, and pancreas. I have seen countless cases that carry misdiagnoses such as Crohn's Disease, colitis, and irritable bowel syndrome when food poisoning was the true underlying cause.

I explained to Karen how anxiety can actually stem from a swollen stomach. A swollen stomach pushes into the esophageal area causing increased pressure. The swelling also impinges upon the vagus nerve, known as "the traveling nerve." The vagus nerve is actually a cranial nerve originating in the brain. It radiates outward traveling to every organ, gland, muscle, and system of the human body. When the vagus nerve is inflamed; anxiety, heartburn, heart attack symptoms, and shortness of breath are just a few of the ensuing symptoms.

I suggested probiotics to restore gut health; digestive enzymes to reduce stomach inflammation; a holistic remedy for salmonella; and an adrenal support to improve strength.

Karen's symptoms improved within one week.

I encourage my patients to become "the keeper of your own body." I educate them about symptoms and their deeper meaning hoping to empower them with the confidence to self-diagnose and treat their own ailments and concerns whenever possible. Karen has taken that advice to heart. As a keeper of her own body she now visits my office twice a year and remains her own good health ambassador by making mindful choices and remaining keenly attuned to her own body.

LOGAN: CAR ACCIDENT INJURIES

LOGAN WAS DRIVING home during a snowstorm one January afternoon. The wind blew so hard that she began to lose control of her vehicle. She swerved hard right to avoid an oncoming truck. Despite her desperate attempts, Logan struck the oncoming vehicle. Windshields were smashed, axles were bent and smoke rolled toward the winter sky. Both engines wheezed. A bloodied and stunned Logan was airlifted to the nearest critical care hospital.

Triage, stabilization, and a series of X-Rays revealed that the fierce impact left Logan with a broken shoulder, a broken femur, numerous fractured ribs, a bleeding spleen, and punctured lungs.

Logan was scheduled for a splenectomy the following morning. Instead, she sought my consultation.

To stop internal bleeding, I recommended two ounces of liquid chlorophyll every hour until morning. Liquid chlorophyll has been found to help even in extreme cases of hemorrhaging. By morning her spleen had healed and her surgery for spleen removal was canceled.

Logan remained under my care for regular chiropractic visits, myofascial release, nutritional support, and Neuro-Emotional Techniques (NET) to help her heal from lasting emotional trauma.

Since her wreck, Logan has continued to heal and thrive. She has since graduated with a degree in nursing and is currently an RN. Logan strives to look at each patient through a broader, more holistic lens. She is interested in furthering her career by becoming a Nurse Practitioner. Logan's outcome and life in general would have been entirely different if she hadn't sought an opinion from a less-traditional medical professional. Logan is both an example and an advocate for living fully by making more mindful self-driven health choices.

RALPH: COMPLICATIONS FROM A PREVIOUS ACCIDENT

RALPH LOVED HIS work in commercial construction. But after years of tearing down dilapidated walls, pouring concrete and hammering steel nails his arm began to throb and tingle. Ralph was referred to a neurosurgeon who performed a battery of X-rays on his neck, shoulders, back and arms. The X-rays revealed that Ralph had several bulging discs in his upper vertebra. The neurosurgeon recommended that Ralph undergo surgery in order to fuse those spinal column bones located in his upper spine. The neurosurgeon strongly felt that surgery was Ralph's only viable road to recovery.

Ralph sought my consultation and treatment prior to committing to the neurosurgeon's recommendation for invasive spinal surgery. As a result, I conducted a complete exam of Ralph's spine and cranium. My examination revealed a misalignment in Ralph's sacral, thoracic, and cervical spine. When vertebra are compromised, as in Ralph's case, the innervating nerves are typically the root causes of associated discomfort. Bearing this information in mind, I suspected that Ralph's arm pain stemmed from his spine's lack of synchronicity.

It's important to note that Ralph had an accident that preceded his arm pain. Three years prior, Ralph suffered a serious blow to the head that led to blindness in his right eye. When I learned of Ralph's prior accident, I became even more convinced that his current condition was directly linked to his past injuries.

The third cranial nerve, the Oculomotor nerve, when not functioning properly, may result in impaired vision. In Ralph's case, the compromised Oculomotor nerve rendered his right eye completely blind.

The accessory nerve, radiating from the fifth and seventh neck vertebra can cause discomfort (pain, numbness, and tingling) in the shoulders, neck, and arms. In order to realign Ralph's spine and cranial bones I recommended both a chiropractic and cranial bone adjustment. Ralph agreed.

Ralph found his job as a construction worker exciting and fulfilling. He feared that arm and shoulder difficulties coupled with his current vision impairment would eventually result in job loss, disability, and saying good-bye to a career that brought him immense joy and satisfaction.

I have treated countless cases in which spinal compression symptoms lie dormant for years before manifesting in pain, numbness, weakness, blindness or other forms of discomfort. Ralph's was another one of these cases.

After the chiropractic and cranial adjustments, Ralph stood up, and circled his arms in the air in order to see if he could sense any shift in his level of discomfort. Not only had the adjustments alleviated Ralph's arm, neck and back pain, but within three weeks the vision in Ralph's right eye was completely restored. For the first time since his accident, Ralph could clearly see.

I have witnessed the immense healing power of such chiropractic and cranial adjustments in literally hundreds of similar and not-so-similar scenarios. The ripple effect of chiropractic care continues to surprise even me after decades of practicing as a licensed Chiropractor.

Ralph and I have remained friends over the years. I am happy to report that he was able to fully resume his beloved career in construction. Possessing a kind and helpful spirit, Ralph is always eager to help me with my household projects from time to time. His vision remains fully restored and his health is intact. As a doctor, nothing brings me more pleasure than bringing a patient back to what brings them joy. In Ralph's case that happiness entails hammering nails, laying tile, and hanging drywall.

NATHAN: STREP

ONE OF MY most memorable experiences was treating a young boy with strep. I was truly humbled by the path in which he came to me. His father informed me that he sought my help because according to his source "I could fix anything." To me, such a ringing endorsement was complicated. Firstly, it is high praise. Secondly, having the high bar of expectation to fix "anything" can actually feel quite stressful.

The father's son, six-year-old Nathan, had been diagnosed with strep throat (caused by infection with streptococcal bacteria) already over a dozen times in his young life. With each diagnosis he was sent home with another round of antibiotics and no clear solution. After thorough testing I discovered that Nathan had a chronic mononucleosis virus. To me, the mono virus was driving the strep.

When a virus lingers the immune system is inherently weakened. The body is then susceptible to bacterial and fungal infections. A recurring bacterial infection means a virus is hard at work.

Nathan was frustrated by his ongoing infection. All he wanted to do was feel better so he could be outside running around kicking the soccer ball like most boys his age. Thankfully, Nathan wouldn't have to wait too long to be back out on the soccer field with his buddies.

I prescribed an adrenal support, an anti-viral support to neutralize the virus, and a probiotic to help rebuild the compromised "good" bacteria in Nathan's gut broken down from long term antibiotics.

Nathan was playing like a champ again within two weeks. In fact, Nathan's dad called me from the car on their way home from our appointment to inform me how much better Nathan was feeling. Last I heard Nathan hasn't used his albuterol inhaler since.

KIMBERLY: RAYNAUD'S SYNDROME AND SCLERODERMA

In over twenty-five years of healthcare practice, I have witnessed some astonishing cases; however, this particular story stands out in the foreground of my memory.

Kimberly, a stunningly beautiful high-energy real estate executive, was diagnosed with Raynaud's Syndrome and Scleroderma. Both of these autoimmune diseases typically have no great outcome. The traditional treatment for Raynaud's Syndrome is steroids, or a combination of an autoimmune suppressant and calcium channel blockers. The side effects of these treatments can be far worse than the disease itself. Kimberly's story illustrates this point beautifully.

Over the span of a month or two Kimberly's hands and feet turned purple and cold-to-the touch. The doctor informed Kimberly that amputation was required within a year's time in order to save her life. Sadly, he explained, that there was just no other option.

I examined Kimberly's hands and feet and immediately wanted to help.

My testing revealed that Kimberly suffered from two infected root canals. I also detected congested lymph nodes located ipsilateral of the previous Root Canal. Kimberly acknowledged that she, in fact, experienced pain in that area of her jaw for many months. At times that pain was unbearable.

After discovering the core cause, I immediately referred Kimberly to a biological dentist. The dentist extracted Kimberly's problem teeth. Shortly after the extraction, I received an SMS photograph of Kimberly's hands and feet from the dentist who performed the procedure. The color had returned to her extremities and according to the dentist her hands and feet were now as warm as toast. My heart sang.

More than 25 million root canals are performed every year in this country.

A tooth with a Root Canal is essentially a "dead" tooth that can become a silent incubator for highly toxic anaerobic bacteria. Under certain conditions these bacteria stealthily enter the bloodstream and cause grave medical conditions. Many of these symptoms are "blind," in extreme cases not rearing their toxic heads until decades later.

Most of these toxic teeth feel and appear unremarkable for long periods. Their quiet origins make their role in systemic disease difficult, perhaps impossible, to trace.

Furthermore; bacteria are captured and destroyed in the context of a healthy immune system. The efficiency of an immune system; however, can be significantly weakened by an accident, illness, or any other bodily or emotional trauma. The human body is susceptible to a myriad of infections without the full function of a robust immune system. Possessing an immune system that seeks-and-destroys pesky bacteria are keys to continued health. Otherwise, free-floating bacteria can ride unencumbered throughout the bloodstream and sneakily set up camp in any new unsuspecting gland, organ, or tissue.

Sadly, the vast majority of dentists are oblivious to the serious extenuating health risks when they perform root canals. Despite the lack of research, The American Dental Association alleges that root canals are proven to be safe though no published work exists to substantiate these claims.

Early in my practice, dentist and friend Dr. John Tate educated me regarding the hidden risks of root canals outlined in George Meinig's 1994 book *Root Canal Cover-up*.

He explained how over a century ago a researcher and dentist discovered that a tooth with a Root Canal is often linked with disease. The dentist, Weston Price, is regarded by many as the greatest dentist of all time. Were it not for his pioneering discoveries many people would continue to suffer from insidious consequences of root canals such as the unnecessary loss of infected teeth and limbs. Kimberly was one of the lucky ones.

Dr. Price gathered evidence regarding the dangers of a Root Canal in his work with rabbits. By transferring human fragments of a Root Canal into a rabbit's bloodstream he discovered that a rabbit would be similarly affected (poor rabbit). For example, he found that transferring fragments from a patient who suffered a heart attack would similarly cause the same result (heart attack) in a rabbit who received those same transplanted fragments.

Nearly every chronic degenerative disease, he found, could somehow be linked to the aftermath of a root canal. The following is an incomplete list of such diseases:

Heart disease
Kidney disease
Arthritis, joint, and rheumatic diseases
Neurological diseases (including ALS and MS)
Autoimmune diseases (lupus and more)

Carrying this idea forward, researcher Dr. Robert Jones suspected a direct correlation between root canals and breast cancer. In a five-year study of 300 breast cancer patients he compiled the following facts:

93 percent of women with breast cancer previously underwent root canals
7 percent had other oral pathologies

In the majority of cases tumors manifested ipsilateral of the root canal or other oral pathologies.

Dr. Jones hypothesized that toxins from infected teeth or jawbones inhibit tumor-suppressing proteins. German physician Dr. Josef Issels reported similar findings. After four decades of practice, Dr. Issels reported that 97 percent of "terminal" cancer patients previously underwent root canals at some point.

If these physicians are correct, cancer prevention may lie primarily in the dentist's chair. Regardless of the origin, a fully functioning immune system is critical in both prevention and treatment of any chronic disease.

Fast forward three years and Kimberly's hands and feet remain intact, healthy and fully functioning. Kimberly is a far cry from the frightened and desperate woman I met in my office years ago at the precipice of having her hands and feet amputated.

AMBER: CHRONIC NECK, BACK AND SHOULDER PAIN

AMBER, AGE 26, complained of chronic neck, shoulder, and back pain. As I examined her I discovered extreme tension in her jaw. I asked Amber if she had a predisposition for grinding her teeth at night. She informed me that her dentist, in fact, had previously diagnosed her with TMJ. She added, according to her dentist, that her teeth were gradually breaking down from this incessant nocturnal grinding. Amber also suffered from poor sleep hygiene due to snoring. Sleeping was not restful by any stretch of the imagination.

I treated Amber using Neuro Integration System and discovered that Amber's nose was slightly misaligned. I asked Amber if she ever suffered from a broken nose. Amazed, she responded "How did you know?"

Amber suffered a broken septum and cracked frontal bone in her forehead several years prior from a car accident. Using NIS, I realigned her nose and reintegrated her brain with the old injury. Amber experienced immediate relief. Literally within seconds, Amber's neck, jaw, and back pain disappeared.

Thirty days later during a follow-up visit, Amber expressed how not only had her insidious pain subsided but how she now slept soundly through the night. Her ability to sleep soundly are the direct benefits of the NIS procedure performed in my office that day. Unbeknownst to Amber, her oxygen intake had been severely compromised from her misaligned septum. For the first time in years, Amber was finally able to get some much needed rest and no longer grinded her teeth.

ANTHONY: CHRONIC ASTHMA

SIX-YEAR-OLD ANTHONY COMPLAINED of shortness of breath and light-headedness for years. According to his mother, Anthony suffered from asthmatic bouts since infancy.

My testing revealed that Anthony suffered from a respiratory syncytial virus since the age of two. Not surprisingly, that was around the same time that Anthony experienced his first trip to the Emergency Room for extreme asthma-like symptoms. Since that time, Anthony had been prescribed antibiotics and later a regimen of steroidal and albuterol inhalers, as well as several antihistamines.

Despite these prescriptions, Anthony continued to struggle.

Anthony's system was likely worn down from years of antibiotics. It's also important to note that over the years of diagnosing and treating upper respiratory issues like Anthony's I've noticed a pattern of weakened adrenal functioning as a result of extended steroidal inhaler use.

In fact, according to renowned cancer researcher Dr. Zach Bush, recovery from just one round of antibiotics can take up to twelve months. After rigorous science and extensive clinical research in his Virginia Clinic, Dr. Bush developed a new group of health products to help expedite the recovery and restoration process.

After my diagnosis I recommended a homeopathic remedy from King Bio, Chronic Viro Reliever, an adrenal support and a probiotic supplement named "Restore."

I have witnessed prompt recovery and restoration from antibiotics in my patients with the use of Restore and hoped for the same outcome for Anthony.

Anthony's breathing improved considerably just a short while after following my recommendations. Fast forward eight years and Anthony remains symptom-free. Now, instead of daily inhalers and antihistamines Anthony maintains respiratory health with routine checkups and chiropractic adjustments.

FREEDA: FIBROMYALGIA

FREEDA SUFFERED FROM pain, muscle tenderness, lack of concentration, and depression. As the primary caregiver for both elderly and ailing parents she frequently felt overwrought and depleted. To seek relief, Freeda sought treatment from a laundry list of doctors. She was diagnosed with fibromyalgia and depression and prescribed an antidepressant, an anti-anxiety medication, and cholesterol and pain medications. Sadly, after years of devoted caregiving, Freeda's parents died just weeks apart.

I met Freeda shortly after her devastating losses. "I loved walking, gardening, and singing in the church choir. I can't do any of these things now. My life is over," she explained while tears streamed down her face.

My examination of Freeda revealed chronic mononucleosis mated with a lingering unresolved emotional issue from her early twenties. Freeda explained how she had been diagnosed with mononucleosis her sophomore year in college. Around the same time Freeda became unexpectedly pregnant and chose to terminate her pregnancy. The stress and duress of both issues impacted Freeda's emotional wellness and the efficiency of her immune system acutely.

Freeda did what most of us do after a crisis, she pulled her life up by the "bootstraps" and did her best to move forward.

Unfortunately, trauma experts explain that unresolved trauma like Freeda's can remain stored in the body until processed carefully under the guidance of a psychotherapist experienced in healing trauma. Pulling ourselves up by the bootstraps doesn't address

our pain and fear. Stored trauma can wreak havoc in many ways. Some of the more extreme symptoms include flashbacks, nightmares, hyper-vigilance and anxiety.

Freeda's life moved forward. She married a man she loved and bore three children. Unfortunately, Freeda hemorrhaged severely during the delivery of her third child. As a result, Freeda was given a full hysterectomy.

A few years after the hysterectomy, Freeda began experiencing severe pain after eating. Tests were performed and it was determined that Freeda needed her gallbladder removed. After having her gallbladder extracted Freeda began to experience extreme anxiety. Consequently, she was prescribed anti-anxiety medication to reduce her anxiety and sleeping medication to help her sleep.

Though Freeda's original diagnosis was chronic mononucleosis my opinion was that her unresolved trauma connected to events of her sophomore year drove her mono. Though symptoms of mononucleosis can clear within two or three weeks, deep emotional scars never completely disappear when left untreated. Emotional wounds like Freeda's can; however, be effectively treated with Neuro Integration System. In my opinion, the most hopeful prognosis for someone like Freeda comes from a combination of correct diagnosis and treatment, neuro emotional clearing using NIS, physical exercise and continued engagement in positive activities.

Freeda now embraces all aspects of her life. She is walking, gardening, and singing in the choir. Doing all of the things that once filled her soul with joy. Freeda continues to focus on emotional and physical maintenance so her body and mind will continue to thrive not merely to survive.

JOHN: STOMACH PROBLEMS

JOHN SUFFERED FROM low energy and stomach problems such as gas, bloating, and a burning sensation after eating certain foods. His primary physician prescribed Prilosec which, according to John, only seemed to make matters worse.

Upon close examination I noticed extensive plaque covering John's teeth. His gums were tender, swollen, red, and bleeding. I discovered an infection in his mouth likely as a result of John's infrequent flossing and brushing. More extensive tests revealed that John's stomach, pancreas, and heart were weak. This is not infrequent. Ingesting bacteria and infection twenty-four hours a day can create extensive internal damage.

I prescribed a liquid called "Great Gums" for John's teeth and gums along with the recommendation for flossing three times a day. A prescription of Bee Propolis was also given for John's lingering infection. Finally, John was provided with a supplement to strengthen the functioning of his heart and adrenal glands.

Two weeks later John returned for his follow-up appointment. He reported a complete absence of prior symptoms. John thanked me with enthusiasm and explained how after years of experiencing a severe lack of energy and listlessness that he now finally felt, "like a million bucks."

ROBIN: ALLERGIES

ROBIN SUFFERED FROM allergies since the age of five. Robin's mother, armed for an allergic reaction, carried an Epipen wherever they went. Though Robin was at risk of anaphylactic shock year round she was especially prone during the spring and fall months when seasonal allergens were floating most densely in the air. Outside of the spring and fall months she was still at risk from an endless list of food allergies.

Robin and her three siblings were frequently sick. They all seemed more susceptible to allergens and illness going around school than the rest of the kids. All four children received several courses of antibiotics when issues would flare. The results were typically ineffective. I suggested Robin and her family receive a Zyto Bioscan.

The ZYTO bioscan relies on galvanic skin response (GSR)—an established technology that measures fluctuations in electrical conductivity of the skin. One familiar application of GSR is lie detector testing.

The ZYTO Hand Cradle measures the user's galvanic skin response and sends that data directly to the ZYTO software for analysis. The GSR data is correlated and compared with Virtual Items in the software database.

Each Virtual Item represents a different physical item. Every time the software introduces a Virtual Item, a corresponding GSR reading is taken by the Hand Cradle. Each new response is measured and tracked in comparison to the GSR baseline reading.

ZYTO's proprietary software analyzes GSR data for patterns of coherence—looking for the ways your GSR readings fluctuate or shift in response to each Virtual Item.

While tracking the GSR data in comparison with each Virtual Item, ZYTO software assigns each Virtual Item a positive or negative value based on the coherence patterns. Positive values indicate Virtual Items that the body is biologically coherent with.

An easy-to-read report is generated that displays a ranking of the Virtual Items that resulted in greater biological coherence. The report can then be used to assist individuals as they make choices to maintain overall health and wellness. We call this whole process biocommunication.

Robin and her three siblings completed a 5 step Zyto Bioscan Allergy Protocol. After more than three years, Robin and her siblings continue to report living a healthy and allergy-free life.

For continued health I recommended that Robin and her entire family take a daily probiotic, and eat locally-grown, organic, non-GMO foods.

For those suffering from chronic allergy symptoms such as an itchy, runny nose, congestion, and sneezing I highly recommend locating a Zyto Technician in your area for diagnosis and treatment.

JIMMY: CHEMOTHERAPY SIDE EFFECTS

I RECEIVED A desperate phone call from a caring son named Jonathan. Jonathan explained that his dad, 49-year-old Jimmy, had been suffering from non-Hodgkin's lymphoma for years. After undergoing months of chemotherapy and radiation, Jimmy had been transferred to the ICU. Jimmy was attached to a respirator and was struggling to breathe. He was suffering from chemotherapy and radiation side effects in conjunction with ramifications from other heavy cancer medications. Jimmy's oncology doctor predicted that he had only four or five days left to live. I explained to Jimmy that I needed some time to process any possible solutions or any way that I could possibly help. Our call ended.

Hearing his four to five-day prognosis was like a kick in the gut. I wondered if any effort to help Jimmy would only be futile and perhaps even negatively impact the quality of his remaining days. Nothing I could do would possibly help him to live longer or alleviate his current symptoms. Attempting to steady my emotions, I cupped my hands to my face and took a series of long deep breaths.

Sensing my distress, my office manager encouraged me to visit Jimmy in the ICU in order to gain a clearer picture of the situation at hand. When I walked into Jimmy's hospital room the situation looked grim. Jimmy's complexion was ashen and a Catholic priest leaned over his hospital bed preparing to perform his Last Rites.

I respectfully asked the priest to allow me a few minutes to further assess Jimmy's condition. The priest nodded. I utilized a technique of Applied Kinesiology and determined that Jimmy's liver, pancreas, kidneys and heart all functioned well. I did; however, conclude that his lung functioning was compromised. More tests revealed a strep infection.

I instructed Jimmy's family to give him a combination of Probiotics, Bee Propolis along with a holistic remedy to help boost his immune system. With Jimmy's diagnosis of non-Hodgkin's lymphoma, I also felt it was essential to prescribe a supplement to help support Jimmy's lymphatic system.

The family informed me that the doctors had identified three holes in Jimmy's lungs either from his cancer or his treatment. This was a critical issue that needed to be addressed immediately. Since infrared light has been known to heal tissue, ligaments, tendons, and tumors I suggested doses of infrared light. I instructed the family to emit the light on his chest at thirty-minute intervals throughout the night. Hopefully the light would permeate his skin and help heal the holes in his chest.

I remember distinctly that the following day was my birthday. I received for my birthday an Infrared light and brought it to Jimmy's hospital room. I recognize now that the gift was not only for Jimmy but for me too. I acknowledged in my heart that the ultimate birthday gift would be if the treatment worked.

I knew chances were slim but I was compelled to try something. At that point, all I had left to do was hope that the family would apply the light treatments and hope for a miracle.

As I exited Jimmy's hospital room I stopped, turned toward his family members and explained that Jimmy was no closer to death then prior to my seeing him. I wrote my personal cell phone number on the back of my business card and left it with the family to "call anytime no matter what time of the day or night."

My heart wrenched, I fully expected to hear of Jimmy's demise sooner than later. Two days passed with no phone call. The following day, Jonathan walked into my office beaming with news. He said the holes in Jimmy's lungs had reportedly healed and, in fact, Jimmy had been discharged from the hospital earlier that day.

I continued to treat Jimmy. We cultivated a close bond. I also felt very connected to his wife Joy and the rest of his family. Connections like these are the reason I became a doctor.

Jimmy lived for another five years. I was at his bedside when he died July 8th, 2010. Joy tells me that his last five years were his most meaningful. She thanked me. We both wept.

Never ever give up hope.

TARA: CARPAL TUNNEL, ALLERGIES

TARA HAD BEEN diagnosed with carpal tunnel syndrome, a painful progressive condition caused by compression of the median nerve in the wrist. She also reported a history of chronic sinus infections and various allergies. Though Tara had one son and craved more children but was unable to become pregnant again. She had previously received treatment for her carpal tunnel syndrome and had been screened for reproductive issues. Her doctors recommended wrist surgery for her carpal tunnel syndrome and fertility drugs to enhance her pregnancy odds.

Tara felt her doctor's orders were extreme and consequently was reluctant to follow through with their recommendation.

A close friend, aware of Tara's reluctance, encouraged her to seek me out for consultation and a second opinion.

My battery of tests revealed that Tara had contracted a virus when she was 12-years old. Though Tara contracted this virus over a decade ago, it continued to affect her hormonal and autoimmune system.

More extensive testing identified the magnitude of her hormonal imbalances, as well as misalignment of her fifth cervical vertebra. I suggested supplements and holistic remedies to negate the virus along with a chiropractic adjustment to alleviate her "carpal tunnel syndrome."

After her adjustment the pain in Tara's wrist vanished immediately. The supplements and holistic remedies also remedied Tara's allergy symptoms. Within three months Tara was pregnant with triplets (without the use of fertility drugs). Today, Tara is a busy

Mom to four beautiful children. Fortunately, she now has the full use of her wrists to cook, fold laundry, and zip up jackets in order to keep up with the demands of her growing family.

CONOR: SCHIZOPHRENIA

CONOR WAS DIAGNOSED with schizophrenia as a young adult. The psychotropic drugs he had been prescribed made him lethargic and negatively impacted his sleep hygiene. After years of taking pills he wanted some alternatives.

Past words of mentor Dr. Theodore Baroody rang in my head. I remember him explaining to me that ninety-five percent of mental disorders directly result from a thyroid imbalance.

I examined Conor using methods of Applied Kinesiology and Neurological Integration System (NIS). My examination revealed that Conor suffered from Hashimoto's encephalopathy. Hashimoto's encephalopathy (also known as steroid-responsive encephalopathy) produces symptoms similar to schizophrenia such as personality changes, aggression, delusional behavior, concentration and memory problems, disorientation, tremors; ataxia, visual hallucinations, seizures, speech problems, insomnia, jerking muscles and overall confusion.

Since the symptoms of HE are similar (almost exact) to a psychological thought disorder HE could easily be misconstrued as schizophrenia.

Though the exact cause of HE is unknown it was first identified in 1966 and is associated with autoimmune thyroiditis. Autoimmune thyroiditis is a chronic inflammatory disorder of the thyroid gland where abnormal blood antibodies and white blood cells mistakenly attack and damage healthy thyroid cells.

Thyroid problems such as Conor's are difficult to diagnose with a blood test. For this reason, it's understandable how Conor's real issue may fly under the radar. Unfortunately, thyroid dysfunctions typically remain undetectable until the thyroid is in a diseased state.

If a person has had a thyroid infection for an extended period, the infection can cross the blood-brain barrier, and cause cerebral inflammation. Symptoms of cerebral inflammation (depending upon where the swelling occurs in the brain) can include weakness, headaches, dizziness, vision loss, lack of coordination and speech impairment.

Symptoms ebb and flow contingent upon the patient's stress level and diet. Since the issue is viral, I have found great success in treating the initial virus.

I suspect that Hashimoto's encephalopathy is one of the most misdiagnosed conditions that continue to fill our Psychiatric hospitals and emergency rooms. Anti-depressants, anti-anxiety medications, and antipsychotic medications, continue to keep those misdiagnosed in the throes of an ineffective mental health system. Erroneous verdicts sentence people like Conor to a lifetime of psychotropic drugs.

It is my opinion that our society continues to stigmatize anyone suffering from a mental illness. We continue to judge through an unsympathetic lens even though science continues to confirm that the source of mental illness rests within the brain. We'd never think to judge someone with diabetes or Crohn's disease; however, when a person is diagnosed with bipolar disorder or schizophrenia we immediately think that they are somehow to blame, that their condition is perhaps a direct result of a defect of character or a sheer unwillingness to try. My hope is that we can change our collective point of view and stop being tone deaf when it comes to mental illness.

Five months after treating Conor's misdiagnosed issue I'm happy to report that he is functioning well and is no longer shackled to a lifetime sentence of medication.

JOSHUA: GRAVES' DISEASE

JOSHUA HAD BEEN diagnosed with Graves' disease. Graves' disease, also known as toxic diffuse goiter, is caused by an overactive thyroid gland. Symptoms include weight loss, fatigue, tremors, irritability, restlessness, insomnia, bulging eyes, excessive sweating, diarrhea, and high blood pressure. Joshua's primary physician prescribed thyroid medication and blood pressure medication. He added that Graves' disease was incurable and that he would have to remain on thyroid medication for the rest of his life. Joshua was 32-years old when he received this diagnosis and the unfortunate forecast of remaining on prescription medication for the rest of his life.

I evaluated Joshua using Neurological Integration System (NIS), a system created by Dr. Allan Phillips. During my evaluation I discovered Joshua's inability to absorb iodine properly. Because of his malabsorption Joshua was suffering from an iodine deficiency.

I educated myself later that evening on the causes and symptoms associated with Graves' disease. I discovered that an inability to absorb iodine is one of the hallmarks of those suffering from Graves' disease. According to the Kahn Institute the brain sends over 100 trillion signals per second to the body. Subsequently, if the iodine signal was "turned off" then Joshua's vital iodine absorption pathway would subsequently shut down. Using Dr. Phillips' NIS system, I reintegrated Joshua's brain's ability to absorb iodine into his system. After three sessions of NIS I asked Joshua to return to his primary physician for follow-up blood work.

Joshua's second round of blood tests indeed confirmed that his "Graves' disease" was in complete remission. Joshua returns to my office for biannual visits to ensure his health is optimal. He no longer carries the burden of taking a lifetime of medication.

MARGARET: SEVERE BACK PAIN

MARGARET CAME TO my office with severe back pain. Three months prior to her visit she slipped and fell on black ice and fractured several ribs. Margaret's recovery was slow. Months later she continued to experience difficulty breathing deep, excruciating pain, and an inability to resume her "normal" daily activities. It's important to note that Margaret's "normal" activities are likely different from most. Margaret's daily regimen consisted of swimming a mile at the pool and walking or running another five on a well-plotted course around her neighborhood.

After her fall, Margaret's primary physician referred her to an orthopedic surgeon. The surgeon examined her X-rays and MRI and recommended that she stop running and even walking all together. According to her physician, Margaret was filled with arthritis. He said her arthritis was so severe in fact that her bones would continue to deteriorate even when doing simple household chores like washing and drying dishes. To someone like Margaret that grim prognosis sounded like a death sentence.

During my evaluation, I discovered that one of Margaret's ribs had healed improperly. The rib was misaligned and as a result cartilage had formed around the rib for repair causing pressure on the thoracic cavity nerves. I knew resetting the rib was imperative. I also knew the process would be excruciatingly painful.

I consulted with fellow chiropractor Dr. Nicholas Wise, known for his bone re-setting experience and expertise. Dr. Nick reset Margaret's rib. The process was painful but the outcome was, according to Margaret, "totally worth it." Within hours, Margaret was literally dancing an Irish jig. Margaret didn't tell me this, I witnessed it with my own eyes. To be fully transparent, I was privy to her jigging because this is my mother's story. Margaret's name is Margaret Keville.

As outlined above my mother is 85-years strong. She came by her strength honestly enough. Born in a small Irish town called Ballyglunin she would be classified as "dirt poor" in every sense of the word. Life was hard and food was scarce. Travelling anywhere meant miles by foot or on the back of a donkey. Drinking water was harvested from a creek a mile away and food was cooked on an open hearth. Though her life was hardscrabble she still mused about the serenity of the rolling Irish hills. She immigrated to the United States when she was only 17-years old chasing the promise of a land whose "streets were lined in gold." Without a quarter in her pocket, she bartered the cost of a ticket for work as a servant in a home of a prominent Long Island family. My young mother slogged, sweated and labored for her hand to mouth existence.

Though time, distance, and life circumstances have kept us apart she reached out to me later in life when she was in pain.

I sometimes wonder if our roles had been in some ways reversed. Having an extensive background in health and wellness, I'd like to think that I played a critical role in modeling healthy living for my age-defying mom. I am happy that I was able to make an impact in that way and utterly grateful that I could relieve her of her suffering. Of course, mom is running, walking, and swimming again. She's training for an upcoming 10K and a marathon later this year. At this point in her recovery my 85-year old mom is back to running circles around me.

GARY: CHRONIC FATIGUE, DEPRESSION

GARY, A 6TH grade Social Studies teacher, couldn't seem to get enough rest. Even though he was logging in more hours of sleep than ever, he continued to feel groggy and weak. Gary struggled every morning just to put his feet on the floor. Some days, the simple act of getting out of bed was literally impossible.

Gary scheduled an appointment with his General Practitioner. Gary's GP subsequently ran a series of tests that were inconsequential. Gary's GP then suggested that, unbeknownst to Gary, he may be struggling with some underlying emotions. At this point in the doctor's decision tree Gary was referred to a psychiatrist in order to treat his suspected subterranean emotions.

The psychiatrist evaluated Gary. Since Gary's symptoms were indicative of depression, he was prescribed Prozac. Within two weeks of taking Prozac, Gary began experiencing panic attacks.

He returned to his psychiatrist and explained the outcome of taking the antidepressant. The psychiatrist responded by writing Gary another prescription this time for anti-anxiety medication.

The prescribed anti-anxiety medication, Xanax, was effective for about four weeks at which time Gary began to experience visual hallucinations, bouts of anger, bouts of sadness, and near panic attacks.

Gary's emotional instability began to take a toll on his job performance and relationship with his kids and wife. His job, marriage, and steady bond with his two children were all starting to unravel.

Gary returned to the psychiatrist again who wrote a different prescription this time to treat Gary's increased symptoms. Gary and his psychiatrist both hoped that his new medication would eliminate his hallucinations, mood swings, and outbursts.

Unfortunately, this round of medication caused physical complications which included gastroesophageal reflux (severe acid reflux), constipation and extreme insomnia. To treat his physical complications Gary was prescribed Prilosec for his acid reflux, stool softeners for his constipation and Ambien for his erratic sleep.

Two years and eight medications later, Gary took the advice of a friend, and having exhausted his options, he finally turned to me for help. My testing immediately revealed that Gary had been struggling with chronic mononucleosis.

When testing for mononucleosis it's important to note that a negative result does not necessarily mean that the body is infection-free. If a test is performed too early or too late in the infection cycle the antibodies may remain undetectable. If symptoms persist I suggest a follow-up test in two weeks to either confirm or rule out the diagnosis.

Infectious mononucleosis, an illness resulting from an infection of the Epstein-Barr virus, is contracted through direct exchange of saliva.

Consequently, it is somewhat accurately referred to as "the kissing disease." Though the disease typically affects teenagers individuals of any age can be infected. The other primary way the virus can spread is by food or beverages sharing with someone who has the illness.

Though mono is typically not fatal it has the ability to wreak serious consequences as illustrated by Gary's case. In addition to fatigue other symptoms of mononucleosis include throat soreness, fever, and a painful skin rash. At times, untreated mononucleosis can develop into strep throat, a sinus infection, even tonsillitis. The most extreme cases can result in an inflamed liver or ruptured spleen. Please note that a ruptured spleen permits large amounts of blood to leak into the abdominal cavity potentially resulting in shock or death.

Adding to the list mono may also produce the following conditions: anemia, thrombocytopenia, heart inflammation, nervous system complications, meningitis, and obstructed breathing due to excessively swollen tonsils.

Typically symptoms will disappear within four to eight weeks. Gary was not so lucky. Below are more specific signs and symptoms of mononucleosis:

SORE THROAT

Mononucleosis usually begins as a minor sore throat. Mono is a real trickster. It may disguise itself as a common cold lasting for weeks instead of days.

FEVER

As with any infection, a fever will persist. Anyone experiencing a fever for more than a few days should seek immediate treatment.

SWOLLEN LYMPH NODES

Located in your groin area, armpits, and neck, lymph nodes are the beholder of vitally important white blood cells. When the body is under attack from bacteria white blood cells increase in number and cause the lymph nodes to swell. Without white blood cells the human body would have no defense against bacteria or viruses.

SWOLLEN TONSILS

In addition to swollen lymph nodes tonsils also swell with inflammation. The condition creates such discomfort that the mono sufferer has difficulty swallowing.

FATIGUE

Extreme fatigue is a hallmark of mononucleosis. The body is already under stress and duress from fighting the bacteria. Heightened body temperature and lack of fluids and food can also add to the level of fatigue. Like Gary, it can feel as if no amount of rest is restorative. Fighting to get out of bed is a definite clue that you may be infected with mononucleosis. In addition to taking antibiotics most doctors will advise mono sufferers to take time off from work or school to properly rest and recuperate.

MUSCLE ACHES

Those who have infectious mononucleosis will often complain of sore and achy muscles. Muscle aches are a secondary symptom of fever, fatigue, and extreme food and liquid deficit.

SKIN RASHES

Doctors typically prescribe antibiotics for undiagnosed mono. Antibiotics do not affect viral infections and they simultaneously kill the good protective bacteria in our gut. When this happens our immune system is weakened. Consequently, the mono virus becomes systemic. This can result in a rash closely resembling the measles and may cover both the body and face. The rash can create immense discomfort and may also be very itchy.

After twenty-five years of experience one of my strongest medical opinions is that antibiotics should only be used as a last resort rather than the first knee-jerk remedy.

HEADACHES

Mild to severe headaches may occur until the infectious mononucleosis is cleared.

RED SPOTS

Check for small, red spots or areas that resemble bruises inside the mouth lining or on the roof of the mouth. The spots may be painful and consequently make eating and drinking difficult.

SORE ABDOMEN

While it is rare individuals with mono may experience soreness in their upper abdomen due to a swollen spleen. The spleen may swell approximately four to 21 days after initial symptoms of the disease appear. Other clues of a swollen spleen include jaundice, a yellowish skin tinge on the body, face, and eyes.

My plan of care for Gary included holistic remedies for mono, Vitamin C and Bee Propolis to boost his immune system, Best Digest to repair the abrasive lining in his stomach from excessive medications, and liquid chlorophyll to repair the spleen. Since mono weakens the adrenal glands I also prescribed an adrenal support.

Gary's energy level returned within two weeks along with the quality of his work and relationships.

Since pharmaceutical drugs each carry their own side-effects, it's important to use extreme caution. The interactive effects of taking multiple medications are highly unpredictable and can vary from person to person. I believe that there is a time and a place in which pharmaceutical drugs can be used appropriately. If a person is in physical or mental crisis then medication can provide a short term solution. Sustained medication when not completely imperative can have harmful consequences.

MICHAEL: AUTISM

I MET MICHAEL for the first time when he was ten years old. He had been diagnosed with autism and the inability to speak when he was just four. Michael had a very low frustration tolerance when playing with others and he did not like to be touched. Because of this, most his days were spent playing video games and watching TV alone in his bedroom.

Michael's backstory is unfortunate. He experienced trauma at a very young age. His biological mother was addicted to methamphetamine and his mother's boyfriend physically and sexually abused him. In the hurricane of her addiction, Michael's Mother was either unaware or didn't care about the daily horror that little Michael was experiencing at the hands of her own boyfriend.

Michael was quickly removed from his Mother's care after the Department of Family and Children Services learned of his abuse. Shortly thereafter, Michael was adopted by a stable and loving family. Michael's new family wanted to help him in any way they could. Helping him to connect with others was a high but necessary hurdle he needed to overcome. With Michael's difficult upbringing we all knew that the road to his recovery would be long.

I conducted a series of intensive examinations and my findings were extensive. My tests revealed that Michael had imbalances of the heart, kidneys, lymphatic system, pancreas, and stomach as well as constipation and chronic anxiety. From a neuro emotional perspective, Michael's bottled up pain and sorrow festered until his body and brain functions ceased developing and began shutting down.

Trauma alters the brain especially in the young, shrinking cognitive areas and increasing the areas on high alert for danger. Trauma sufferers can continue to experience a heightened state of dread and panic. Michael's early life experiences likely impacted his normal growth and brain development.

Using Neuro Integration System, I slowly began to clear and balance Michael's body. When I cleared residual emotions of his broken heart, created by the abuse I observed his eyes tearing. The tears gently streamed down his cheeks involuntarily. Within minutes Michael began to talk, smile, laugh, and even clap his hands.

The Adverse Childhood Experiences (ACEs) Study is a well-known research study conducted by Kaiser Permanente health maintenance organization and the Centers for Disease Control and Prevention.

This study directly links adverse childhood experiences to future health and social problems as an adult. ACEs researchers follow participants for many years in order to gather information and compile significant information to determine the long term cause and effects of early trauma like Michael's. Results conclude that a person's cumulative ACEs score strongly correlates to numerous health, social and behavioral problems as well as substance abuse and process addiction disorders.

Therapies such as Neurological Integration System, Craniosacral Therapy, energetic medicine (acupuncture, yoga, and kinesiology) and neurofeedback, are often utilized in cases like Michael's as methods for trauma-resolution. My patients have found much relief from such methods. Michael has benefitted greatly from the work we've done together. The boy who once never uttered a word now, according to his adopted Mother, "hasn't stopped talking!" Michael's language skills have soared. He loves to read books about trains and space as well as graphic comics. Perhaps most importantly, Michael has a new friend. He has learned how to be present and aware with another young boy his age. Together they play side by side.

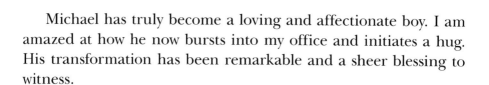
Michael has truly become a loving and affectionate boy. I am amazed at how he now bursts into my office and initiates a hug. His transformation has been remarkable and a sheer blessing to witness.

RANDY: LOW BACK PAIN

RANDY COMPLAINED OF chronic low back pain, difficulty sitting, walking, and standing. He previously received treatment from a range of health care professionals including chiropractors, a physical therapist, massage therapists, and an orthopedic doctor. When I met Randy he was slated to undergo back surgery with an orthopedic surgeon. His surgery was three weeks away.

During my palpation exam, I noticed two scars in the inguinal area near Randy's hips. Randy reported that he had inguinal hernia repairs on each hip and the scars were a result of his surgery. Alarm bells rang. Though the scar tissue existed on Randy's hips (on the front of his body) he experienced pain in his back. The scars were suspected culprit of Randy's pain. Scar tissue can create tightness and discomfort permeating through to the opposite side of the body and traveling upward or downward as Randy's case illustrates.

Since scar tissue in effect shrinks "like Saran Wrap" over time the discomfort created by the tight pull may not surface until years later. I utilized Barnes Myofascial Release in order to alleviate the tightness of Randy's scar tissue. After the procedure he felt his back pain slowly subside. Another 30 minutes passed and his pain disappeared completely. Over the last eight years Randy returns like clockwork for his annual check-ups. I monitor any changes in Randy's scar tissue. His flexibility remains nimble and his overall health is excellent.

KATLYN: SEIZURES

Two-year old Katlyn began experiencing seizures shortly after receiving her DPT vaccine. Her concerned parents were desperate to find a treatment for her violent attacks. I examined Katlyn using Applied Kinesiology and palpation and discovered vaccination toxins that included mercury poisoning. Mercury, a naturally occurring yet dangerous heavy metal, is commonly used in the manufacture of vaccines. When it is breathed in as a vapor or absorbed through the blood it can cause mood swings, headaches, weakness, muscle twitching, insomnia, nervousness and irritability.

I used a holistic remedy to thoroughly remove the mercury and other toxins from Katlyn's body. As a result, I informed Katlyn's parents to expect a massive bowel movement during which time the toxins poisoning her blood would be eliminated. After that the seizures would end. As expected, Katlyn did purge the poisons. Fourteen years have passed and Katlyn has remained healthy and seizure-free.

SARAH: LUPUS

SARAH WAS A sickly child and continued to struggle with health issues her entire life. Sarah was diagnosed with lupus and became my patient at the age of thirty-two.

Systemic lupus erythematosus, referred to as SLE or lupus, is a chronic disease that causes inflammation, pain and swelling. Lupus is actually a constellation of symptoms and its etiology (cause) is unknown. Its wide range of symptoms mimics many other diseases and illnesses.

Consequently, lupus is also referred to as "the great imitator." Because of overlapping symptoms lupus is frequently misdiagnosed.

In addition to affecting the skin and joints, it can affect other organs in the body such as the kidneys, the pleura (tissue lining) in the lungs, the brain, and the heart (pericardium). Most patients experience fatigue, skins rashes, painful and swollen joints and fever.

Lupus flares oscillate from mild to serious. Most patients experience periods when the disease is completely dormant. These symptom-free periods are actually referred to as "remission." Periods of remission can be followed by an intense flare up of extreme and painful symptoms. As of this writing, neither a cause nor a cure for lupus has been identified. Lupus is treated typically with steroids. Unfortunately, long-term steroid use can have extreme and sometimes life threatening consequences.

Testing revealed that Sarah suffered a traumatic experience when she was seven-months old while still developing in her Mother's womb.

As far as Sarah knew, nothing significant happened during her Mother's nine-month pregnancy that would be classified as traumatic. One phone call to her mother revealed a different story. Sarah's mother explained that she in fact experienced her greatest life trauma while pregnant with Sarah. Her mother explained that when she was exactly seven-months pregnant her brother committed suicide. Sadly, Sarah's mother was the one who found her brother dead. Though Sarah's mom was thrilled to be pregnant with Sarah, losing her brother in this heart-wrenching way cast a dark shadow over Sarah's mother's soul and subsequently her pregnancy.

Now we knew the exact cause of Sarah's trauma. A developing baby in its mother's womb experiences the exact same feelings and emotions as the mother since there is no emotional boundary between mother and baby. In light of this information, I now understood that baby Sarah's system had been drenched in stress hormones during a very critical stage of her development. Baby Sarah came into this world already steeped in fight- flight-faint response hormones.

Marred by brain and chemical changes produced by trauma, Sarah's body never had a chance to recuperate. Sarah's life had been plagued by illness, disease and discomfort since birth. It seemed as if, according to Sarah, "The older I get the sicker I become."

I advised Sarah to take a series of nutritional supplements to help reset her nervous system. Holistic remedies for shock include flower essences, adrenal support, probiotics, and minerals. Within a few months of our initial appointment, even small traces of lupus were undetectable in Sarah's blood.

THE EFFECTS OF EARLY TRAUMA

Babies and toddlers are totally dependent upon their primary caregivers for food, safety, and shelter. Loving reassurance expressed through a primary caregiver's warmth, soothing verbal tones, consistent presence, nurturance, and accurate emotional mirroring helps infants to become securely attached. When a young mother experiences trauma of her own she is less able to provide these necessary building blocks. Without the nurturing children can become fraught with emotional attachment issues. An overall lack of normalcy in the home creates uncertainty and affects a child's ability to cope and develop. Here are some examples:

Emotional issues like feeling overwhelmed, fear, sadness, and shock affecting their parents or primary caregiver.

Periods of separation from parents or primary caregiver – for example; absences due to injury, mental illness, substance abuse, incarceration, trauma or other factors that create absence. The impact in these cases are twofold: 1) the infant or child experiences distress due to the absence of the parent and 2) the distress over the insecurity of having to manage their own feelings without the understanding and nurturing of their parents **or** primary caregiver. A condition of complex trauma can develop from chronic or long-term exposure to overwhelming emotional trauma in cases of domestic emotional abuse, physical and sexual abuse.

The general stress and/or sensory overload of the household – babies and toddlers are highly affected by noise, distress, and chaos (parents fighting, barking dogs, strangers coming and going, etc.).

Any other disruption or outside influence that prevents, halts, or disrupts the sensitive and vitally important bonding stage. A child is left susceptible to addiction, mental illness, and extreme relationship difficulties if a bond with the primary caregiver is not cemented in early life.

Simply put, if the family system or primary caregiver is stressed then the baby is stressed.

ANN: TINGLING ELECTRICAL SHOCKS

ANN WAS BITTEN by a copperhead snake while gardening in 2012. She immediately reported to the emergency room after the bite. The ER doctor treated the wound topically then explained that there was nothing else he could do to help with any possible residual effects. He wrote a dual prescription for anti-anxiety and antidepressant to help with the emotional aftermath of the snake bite trauma and discharged her from his care.

Ann's symptoms persisted. She continued to experience a tingling "electric shock" sensation throughout her entire body along with difficulty breathing and nausea. Additional snake bike symptoms can include vomiting, blurred vision, sweating and salivating, and numbness in the face and limbs.

A mutual colleague referred Ann to me to address her continued symptoms and concerns. Bearing in mind complex nature of snake bites I decided to reach out to my mentor, Dr. Ted Baroody, for consultation. Once in the system, he explained, snake venom can linger in the body for month's even years after the bite. Because of this Dr. Ted advised me to create a homeopathic remedy to allow her body to eliminate the snake venom.

Ann closely followed my instructions for taking her energetic remedy. Approximately one week later she returned to my office for a follow-up visit. She was symptom-free. Ann thanked me and expressed relief. She wondered if the uncomfortable sensation would have ever disappeared if she hadn't sought my help.

BILL: HEAVY METAL POISONING

BILL ORIGINALLY CAME to my office inquiring about treatment for his emphysema. Over the years I have learned to be respectfully skeptical especially when it comes to issues related to the upper respiratory system. Consequently, I conducted extensive neurological testing in order to rule out possibilities other than emphysema.

Based on these new findings I asked Bill if he had ever been exposed to heavy metals derived from fossils fuels or plants. He explained that he had sustained exposure during his work as a pharmaceutical chemist. He outlined his work in detail by explaining how the pharmaceutical industry paid him to duplicate naturally occurring plants using petrochemicals and heavy metals.

I was shocked by the extent of Bill's frequent contact with heavy metals and other potentially harmful substances. Since Bill worked as a pharmaceutical chemist for over thirty years his body had likely absorbed thirty years' worth of such poisons.

I created a remedy to help neutralize the effects of Bill's heavy metal exposure. I also recommended Free Breath, an herbal remedy by Dr. Ted Baroody to help detoxify Bill's lungs.

Within a few weeks, Bill showed no signs or symptoms of emphysema.

Bill was my patient for over 15 years. . .

Bill shined with love. He always wore a smile and was one of my most outspoken supporters. Bill encouraged others stranded in medical limbo to seek my help, "Well if Dr. Kate can't figure it out, no one can," he'd say.

Bill witnessed some of life's most unspeakable atrocities. It wasn't until later in life that he began to divulge some of the details of his work as a Military Intelligence Officer in World War II. He began to tell his wife and three grown children how he performed many secret missions during this dark chapter of human history. Some of those missions entailed providing aid and relief to Holocaust prisoners. Though undoubtedly relieved to finally express the emotional load he'd been carrying, Bill's body eventually wore down. He remained kind and charismatic until death, despite the emotional shrapnel I know he carried.

BOBBIE: CHRONIC SHOULDER PAIN

BOBBIE WAS PLAGUED with chronic left shoulder pain. In fact, she could barely lift her arm and shoulder due to the insidious discomfort. Her doctors speculated that she would likely need shoulder replacement surgery. I evaluated Bobbie's left shoulder and discovered the existence of a significant amount of scar tissue. She informed me that she had a pacemaker surgically inserted a few years prior. Though she didn't suspect any connection, Bobbie further explained that her pain developed approximately 12 months after the implantation.

To help loosen the restricting scar tissue I utilized Barnes Myofascial scar tissue technique. After a few treatments, Bobbie's pain dissipated and she regained full range of motion of her left arm.

Bobbie returns biannually to receive her scar tissue treatments. She continues to thrive. This story illustrates the impact that past surgeries and procedures can have on present day health. It's important to remember that even a small surgical procedure can have future consequences. Bearing this information in mind, it's important to share your full medical history with doctors. Though it may seem unrelated the human body is a complex web of overlapping systems. Like dominos every change in the body elicits another reaction.

BRENDA: GALLBLADDER CONGESTION

BRENDA WAS DIAGNOSED with gallbladder congestion. When a gallbladder is congested it slows the gallbladder's storing and release of bile as well as hinders the bile from traveling from the liver to the intestines. Gallbladder congestion may be a prelude to the excruciatingly painful condition of gallstones. An ultrasound revealed the true state of Brenda's gallbladder. Ninety percent of her gallbladder was blocked; consequently, her doctor recommended gallbladder extraction. Brenda lived paycheck to paycheck and didn't have extra money for healthcare let alone a surgery of this magnitude. Financing a procedure like this would have literally forced Brenda into bankruptcy.

Brenda asked me if there was any cost-effective treatment that would help. She was willing to try anything within her grasp that might improve her condition and to help save her gallbladder.

The gallbladder is a small organ that stores bile, an alkaline fluid that aids digestion by helping to breakdown fats, proteins, and sugars. Though the gallbladder is vital the medical field frequently dismisses it as unnecessary. In my opinion the gallbladder should not be treated as a spare part because our system is greatly weakened without it. A weakened or unhealthy gallbladder can lead to Multiple Sclerosis, arthritis, cancer, Alzheimer's or other diseases.

To help Brenda's condition I recommended an organic drink. The product, Greens First, is blended with water and consumed twice a day.

Brenda returned to my office 30 days later. She informed me that her follow-up ultrasound revealed no stones and no congestion. Her gallbladder was now healthy and fully-functioning. The drink completely restored her gallbladder to mint condition. Brenda was also relieved from the stress of possible financial ruin.

KATHERINE: CHRONIC NECK PAIN

KATHERINE SUFFERED FROM extreme neck pain. Her doctor explained that she had degenerative disc disease and that surgery would be required in order to fuse the vertebra in her neck. Katherine was relatively young. She was a robust, active, yoga instructor and mother of two young children. Degenerative disc disease is much more common in people over the age of 60. To me, her diagnosis did not seem accurate.

At the time I had just studied Dr. Allan Phillips' Neuro Integration System. Dr. Allan's system includes a gout protocol. Gout is a type of arthritis caused by a defective metabolism which leads to a buildup of uric acid. Acute pain, redness, and joint tenderness occur episodically from chalkstone deposits. Gout is most commonly found in the smaller bones of the feet or ankles though less common gout can actually occur in any joint.

After several unsuccessful attempts to relieve Katherine's neck pain through other holistic methods I decided to implement Dr. Phillip's gout protocol. I treated Katherine with the protocol then advised her that her system may require up to three weeks in order to properly reabsorb the excess uric acid through the digestible proteins.

Katherine contacted me about two weeks after her treatment. She was elated. She said for the first time in eight long years that she was pain-free for three consecutive days.

One of the lessons in this story is the importance of continued learning. As a seeker of healthcare related knowledge I am always struck at how quickly I am presented with an opportunity to implement a freshly learned concept, skill, or technique. As Benjamin Franklin wrote, "An investment in knowledge pays the best interest." Had I not attended Dr. Phillip's seminar just a few weeks' before Katherine's visit, her proper diagnosis may have remained beyond my reach. Constant learning pays handsome dividends regardless of profession.

CECIL: CHRONIC BACK PAIN, DEPRESSION

IT WAS JUST another busy Tuesday at the office. I briefly looked out the window at the trees outside and caught a glance of their changing colors. I always loved that time of year when the leaves changed from the summer to their autumnal palate. The colors seemed to give me a boost of energy. Since I had a waiting room full of patients and I was again feeling energized I decided to skip lunch and work all the way through until my last patient.

My next appointment was with a man named Cecil. Cecil was in his early eighties and wheelchair bound due to a serious work-related fall. Cecil never fully recovered. A man who worked hard all of his life was now trapped in a wheelchair. The confinement took its toll. Cecil suffered from chronic back pain, listlessness and depression. By the time he came to my office Cecil had lost his will to live.

Cecil stood nearly 7 feet tall. It required three of us to raise Cecil from his wheelchair and stretch him out on my chiropractic table. Cecil's skin tone was an unhealthy grey. His breathing was shallow and his energy ebbed low.

I palpated his spine and discerned that several of Cecil's thoracic vertebra and ribs were misaligned. Cecil's doctors had prescribed a variety of pain medications, blood pressure medications, cholesterol medications, and a high dose of antidepressant to help him cope.

I adjusted Cecil's thoracic spine. At the moment of his adjustment, Cecil let out a loud shriek then immediately passed out. My office manager was in the next room. Startled, she ran into the examination room to assist. My office manager and I both called out Cecil's name over and over while simultaneously tapping his arms hoping to restore his consciousness. Nothing worked. We looked at one another in utter horror wondering if he was dead.

After about a minute or two Cecil finally regained consciousness. At the moment of his restored consciousness he gasped taking in a very large breath. Cecil looked around the room as if to steady himself. He lifted himself up from the table then looked directly into my eyes. I saw tears begin to form. It was clear to me that Cecil cried because he knew that his life would be different from that moment forward. After years of being confined to a wheelchair Cecil was finally liberated.

After completing a thorough physical exam to ensure that Cecil had fully recovered from the day's dramatic event we scheduled a follow-up appointment a few months away. Cecil returned through the waiting room full of patients. The once sickly ashen-skinned man who arrived in a wheelchair walked out with little assistance with a renewed glow and zest for life. I imagine that everyone sitting in that waiting room was just as astonished as my office assistant and I were that day. Don't ever let anyone tell you that miracles don't happen. One happened to Cecil on a typical Tuesday afternoon around 2 o'clock at my office in Spartanburg South Carolina.

DENNIS: CHRONIC SKIN PROBLEMS

DENNIS SOUGHT TREATMENT from a half a dozen doctors within a hundred-mile radius. He suffered from a raspberry red rash that covered the skin on both of his legs. The rash was extremely itchy, uncomfortable, and distracting. Though it was in the middle of Carolina's sweltering summer Dennis was uncomfortable wearing shorts and making his legs visible.

Dennis received a myriad of diagnoses from his variety of doctors. Some of them included psoriasis, eczema, and seborrheic dermatitis. Dennis received no relief from the multitudes of creams, anti-inflammatory drugs, and antihistamines he was recommended.

By means of Holographic Health System, I discovered that Dennis had none of the diagnoses previously named. Dennis, in fact, was experiencing a severe attack of systemic poison ivy and oak. The insidious poisonous sap is found in nearly every part of the plant including the stem, leaves, and roots. After contact the skin develops an instant blistering skin irritation. The sap definitely found its way into Dennis's system.

The poisons had been absorbed into his bloodstream and were likely being "recycled" and reappearing even after extended periods of dormancy. I have observed poison ivy rash reoccurring periodically throughout the year particularly in times of severe stress in several other patients or after periods of extended dormancy.

Steroids are the typical course of treatment. In all cases; however, sustained steroid use suppresses the immune system and consequently drives the poisons deeper into the nervous system.

When the body is compromised in this way it is unable to eliminate poisons, viruses, bacteria, or other toxins. This can result in other skin eruptions such as fungus, hives, or warts. A deep detoxification is required in order to fully restore skin and body health.

I provided Dennis with King Bio homeopathic remedies specifically engineered to address the imbedded poison ivy and oak. Additional supplements were given to boost his immune system and calm his nervous system. I cautioned Dennis that his symptoms might spike before finally clearing.

Within two days, Dennis' wife sent me a picture of his legs. As predicted, the rash had intensified. "Bravo!" I responded. "The rash is finally leaving his body. Better out than in!" Dennis's legs were completely devoid of rash a few weeks later. Unbeknownst to Dennis, he had been walking around with a poisoned system for a long time. Though it took over a year to completely heal, the most severe symptoms dissipated within weeks. Years have passed and Dennis is back to wearing shorts again. His uncomfortable, inflamed, rash has never returned.

MARIA: GRAND MAL SEIZURES

MARIA SUFFERED FROM a history of grand mal seizures. She couldn't walk and her medications seemed to be making her symptoms worse. Her husband Jimmy was desperate. Feeling particularly hopeless, he shared Maria's story with a compassionate person he met one day in the line at the drugstore. Turns out, that compassionate person was a patient of mine. The following morning, I received a phone call from Jimmy. He explained that he had been referred to me by a current patient.

I agreed to see Maria the next day.

Unable to walk, Jimmy carried Maria in his arms. He laid her delicately at the center of my examination table. I performed a battery of tests in order to rule out or confirm a constellation of possibilities. After extensive testing it was clear that Maria's cranium was severely misaligned.

I treated Maria's misalignment with craniosacral therapy. Due to the severity of her misalignment the procedure took over two hours. At one point during therapy, Maria experienced a seizure on my table. The seizure experience was terrifying for Maria and her husband. I assured them that, though frightening, this would be the last seizure she would likely ever have. Fifteen years have passed and Maria has remained seizure-free.

Craniosacral therapy (CST) is a gentle, hands-on approach that releases deep tensions and restrictions in the soft tissues surrounding the central nervous system. CST was pioneered by physician John Upledger. It has been effective in the treatment of a wide range of physical and emotional problems and dysfunctions associated with pain. This gentle, noninvasive form of bodywork targets the bones of the head, spinal column, and sacrum. The release of compression subsequently alleviates stress and pain.

This less traditional approach is radically different from the steroidal treatment typically used to alleviate compression and swelling of the brain and spinal cord.

Short-term effects of steroid use include sodium retention-related weight gain and fluid accumulation, hyperglycemia, glucose intolerance, hypokalemia, gastrointestinal upset and ulceration, mood changes ranging from mild euphoria and insomnia to nervousness, restlessness, mania, catatonia, depression, delusions, hallucinations, and even violent behavior.

Reported long-term effects include metabolic changes, dilation of capillaries, easy bruising, thinning of skin, hirsutism or virilism (appearance of secondary opposite-sex sex characteristics), impotence, menstrual irregularities, peptic ulcer disease, cataracts and increased intraocular pressure/glaucoma, myopathy, osteoporosis, and vertebral compression fractures.

Though craniosacral therapy is most widely used to decrease stress from chronic injuries, after twenty-five years of practice I have found craniosacral therapy to be an effective treatment option with many other conditions and symptoms. Maria's case demonstrates this point beautifully.

PAT: CHRONIC HIP PAIN

PAT SUFFERED FROM chronic pain in his right hip. His doctor told him he would eventually need hip replacement surgery, but was instructed to hold off until the pain was unbearable. I adjusted Pat's hip approximately four times a year. Pat drives approximately 200 miles a day and I knew the stress and duress of being behind the wheel for such an extended period of time must have great impact and resulting pain.

After his last hip adjustment, I followed Pat out to the parking lot in order to observe how he lifted himself into the driver's side of his car. I speculated that the way he raised himself into the car was inducing pain. I didn't notice any irregularity that would create discomfort. I scratched my head in wonder.

Then one day, Pat mentioned in passing that he had been diagnosed with gout. This was the missing link.

Gout is a form of arthritis caused by excess uric acid in the bloodstream. The symptoms of gout result from the formation of uric acid crystals in the joints. Though gout most commonly affects the joint in the base of the big toe it can appear in any joint.

With this critical piece of information in hand, I performed Dr. Allan Phillips' NIS gout protocol. I received a text from Pat a few hours after our session. He reported no hip pain and full range of motion. The complications of gout can be both undetectable and serious. Bearing this information, I rule out gout in complicated cases while moving through my diagnostic decision tree. More often than not the process of elimination eventually leads me to a correct diagnosis.

THERESA: PARTIAL PARALYZATION

THERESA CAME TO me complaining of neck pain. She had been diagnosed with Multiple Sclerosis a decade prior and the complete left side of Teresa's body was paralyzed. She relied on a walker to get to her doctor's appointments, go to church and the grocery store. Though the walker allowed for some mobility her left leg was completely limp and continued to drag behind as she moved from place to place.

In addition to the chronic pain, Theresa had little to no range of motion in her neck. I inquired about past surgeries. She explained how she was diagnosed with breast cancer a decade earlier and as a result had a complete mastectomy of her left breast. I discovered scar tissue where the breast had been removed.

I began using Barnes Myofascial Release on the left breast area to release the pressure from the underlying tightened fascia. During the procedure Theresa felt a tingling sensation followed by throat pressure. Then, she began to cough and gag. We took breaks during the process allowing Theresa to steady her breath.

The procedure continued. I worked cautiously to gently break up the residual scar tissue. Gradually, Theresa reported the sensation of blood flow returning. She noticed it first in her left foot, then her left hip, then her left arm.

Theresa slowly regained some movement in her once frozen limbs. The procedure was so successful that she urged to stay longer in order to receive the full benefit of the treatment that day. Obliging her request, I proceeded to work on her scar tissue delicately and with great caution.

Three hours passed. My hands began to cramp but I was determined to release this woman from the bondage of paralysis.

When the procedure was finally complete the sensation, movement, and range of motion in Theresa's once paralyzed body was now fully restored. Theresa walked out of my office without the assistance of her walker.

Theresa's diagnosis of Multiple Sclerosis was obviously incorrect. I surmised that the scar tissue from Theresa's breast removal wrapped around her brain stem and caused lower and upper motor paralysis. Fifteen years later Theresa continues to live an active life unencumbered by paralysis and neck pain.

BETSY: CHRONIC ELBOW PAIN

BETSY CALLED MY office in the morning stating she had been awake all night from chronic elbow pain. She made an emergency appointment to see me later that afternoon. She explained that she had considered making a chiropractic appointment for this condition earlier but was dissuaded by her friends who insisted that a chiropractor would only make matters worse.

I discovered a scar on Betsy's left wrist and left elbow. She explained that she had surgery for carpal tunnel syndrome a few years prior. Carpal tunnel is rooted in a misalignment of the neck vertebra. Cutting the nerves in the wrist can provide only temporary relief. If the deeper issue remains unaddressed then symptoms will reoccur over time.

Betsy also informed me that she was unable to turn her neck allowing her to look behind her while driving. Instead, she was forced to turn her entire body to assess traffic. To me, that was the likely origin of her wrist problems.

Every vertebra in the spinal column should move in eight directions, and the first vertebra referred as the "Atlas" should move in twelve directions. When joints are not moving optimally then residual problems extend to every organ, gland, limb, and blood vessels, effectively every part of the body.

I performed a chiropractic adjustment to correct the misalignment in Betsy's neck, followed by treatment with Barnes Myofascial Release in order to loosen and free the scar tissue resulting from her previous wrist surgery.

Betsy remains without elbow pain, and her range of motion in her neck is now fluid. The demands of her job working with abused children are no longer impacted by her physical pain. Betsy is one of the most compassionate people I know. Helping helpers like Betsy gives my work even greater purpose. I know that by keeping Betsy healthy she is able to continue with her important work providing support, comfort, and encouragement for others which is very gratifying.

Though I believe a greater understanding is impending I am still astonished by the ongoing stigmatization of chiropractic science. Most of the stigma is rooted in miseducation.

The work of chiropractors is often mischaracterized. We do not "crack" bones. We do; however, gently shift them back into position. The "popping" or "cracking" noise that results is not from the popping or cracking of the actual bone. The sound emitted is caused from the healthy release of gasses accumulated between the compressed joints.

Part of me wonders if the perpetuation of such negative stereotypes is part and parcel of a larger issue. As I commented in my Introduction, I imagine that the powerfully influential and lucrative pharmaceutical industry is not likely to allow alternative methods to cut into their profits. My experience has been that more holistic practitioners are less revenue-driven and more solution-driven. I have witnessed too many success stories like Betsy's to rationally dismiss the benefits of alternative holistic methods.

MELISSA: URINARY TRACT INFECTIONS

MELISSA SUFFERED FROM chronic urinary tract infections (UTI) and vaginal infections for over 20 years. She had been taking antibiotics multiple times a year yet continued to suffer. Melissa was fatigued, depressed, and tired of living.

My testing revealed an evidence of trauma that likely occurred when Melissa was around seven-years old. I probed with compassion asking Melissa about a past event that may register as trauma. Overcome with emotion, Melissa tearfully revealed that she had been molested by her uncle at that time. The event was terrifying yet she told no one.

Bestselling author, radio show host, healer, and cancer survivor Louise Hay carefully outlines diseases, their symptoms and emotional origins in her landmark book You Can Heal Your Life (Hay House, 1984).

Hay traces the emotional origins of bladder complications such as Melissa's urinary tract infection to anger felt for a person of the opposite sex. Using Hay's framework would provide a clear explanation for Melissa's recurring health issues.

Children of sexual trauma are left emotionally maimed. Suppressing their experience by not telling a supportive adult further complicates the trauma. Melissa's perpetrator threatened her promising "bad things will happen if tell you anyone." Without a fully developed prefrontal cortex (where we make decisions and find solutions) the young brain is unable to think of alternatives such as report the incident to the police, tell mom, or inform a teacher.

The body and subconscious mind continues to hold on to the trauma. The trauma festers and is often expressed in a physical or disease-like manner.

In Melissa's case her trauma manifested as a chronic urinary tract infection.

I prescribed a UTI holistic remedy created by King Bio for Melissa's physical symptoms, along with Best Digest. I also implemented Holographic Health techniques to begin to address her deep emotional wounds.

Melissa has been free of physical complications for over five years. Holographic Health allowed the emotional trauma of her past experience to be resolved. The memory will always be there, but the effect on her physical health is eliminated.

KATIE: POSTPARTUM DEPRESSION

KATIE HADN'T SLEPT in over a week. She cared for a newborn baby and a three-year old daughter. She reported fatigue, anxiety, lack of appetite, even visual hallucinations symptoms all consistent with postpartum depression.

I evaluated Katie using Neuro Integration System. My evaluation revealed significant thyroid, spleen, pancreas, and adrenal imbalances. I also detected inflammation in Katie's brain.

At that time my initial assumption would typically be a diagnosis of Hashimoto's Encephalitis. My years' of experience; however, told me a deeper issue existed. So, I continued to remain open to other potential causes and diagnoses. Regardless, I began treating Katie using NIS.

After the first visit, Katie reported that her hallucinations subsided. Her sleeping and eating hygiene also improved significantly.

After two more visits Katie reported feeling completely rested and "back to my old self" feeling light-hearted and playful.

Most "postpartum depression" symptoms are treated with antidepressants and anti-anxiety and sleeping medications. The combination of these drugs can produce extreme side effects like the ones Katie originally reported. Today I'm still uncertain about Katie's actual diagnosis. I do think that postpartum depression may have indeed impacted a deeper issue.

Though I remain curious in my profession I don't need all the answers to be effective. The goal is to restore every patient to health regardless of the speculated diagnose or course of treatment. As long as my patients leave my office happier and relieved of their symptoms then I am satisfied with my role and their outcome.

Katie has been living a successful, content, and "holistic lifestyle" for many years. Katie concluded that treating her symptoms with drugs would only exacerbate her symptoms and potentially cause additional health problems. Katie, her husband, and children are very healthy to this day. Katie is an economist, teacher, and successful book author. Her most recent book is called "Atheist to Enlightenment in Thirty Days".

JACK: HIP AND KNEE PAIN

JACK HAD SURGERY on both knees five years prior to his first visit with me. Now he suffered from hip and knee pain. Jack explained that his doctors recommended a double hip replacement because his hips were gradually "breaking down."

I closely examined Jack's ankles and feet and immediately noticed misaligned bones. I asked Jack if he had previously suffered any sports injuries. He acknowledged that he had, in fact, sprained both ankles multiple times while playing competitive basketball in high school and college.

I immediately adjusted the bones in Jack's feet. His hips were not dislocated they were both just slightly misaligned from the acetabulum, more commonly known as "hip sockets."

Since scar tissue can create problems years after surgery I also treated his residual scar tissue from previous surgeries using Barnes Myofascial Release technique. Scar tissue can cause hidden complications. Scar tissue develops beneath the skin. This tissue, called fascia, looks similar to cheesecloth and behaves similar to plastic wrap.

Following surgical stitching or suturing, the outside fascia becomes shortened. In time, the fascia will twist and may potentially entrap arteries, veins, organs, glands, and muscles. Because of this "tightening" I always recommend treatment by a Barnes Myofascial Therapist or a Neuro Integration Practitioner after surgery.

Jack's hip and knee pain has been alleviated. Additionally, he was able to avoid undergoing a double hip replacement.

GAFFNEY: DEPRESSION, ANGER

GAFFNEY CAME TO my office depressed, angry, sick, and frustrated. She reported yearly episodes of strep throat, chronic depression, no will to live, and a bleak outlook of the future. It's also important to note that Gaffney suffered extensive childhood trauma for years by a family friend.

Originally, I discovered chronic incidents of strep pneumonia originating nearly from birth. Gaffney confirmed that she, in fact, had almost died from pneumonia as an infant. Gaffney spent most of her childhood and adult life on frequent regimens of antibiotics and antihistamines. She had also been prescribed a multitude of anti-depressants, anti-anxiety medications, by many doctors.

I prescribed Gaffney remedies for her lifelong strep which included a variety of minerals, digestive enzymes, and an adrenal support. I'm thrilled to share that Gaffney has reported no symptoms of strep or any other of the above listed ailments. Her lifelong need for antibiotics has disappeared.

Shortly thereafter, in order to further treat residual traumatic symptoms, I suggested that Gaffney try Neurofeedback. Experiencing daily hyper vigilant states of flight, fight, or freeze is not uncommon for trauma survivors and I was excited by the opportunity to help Gaffney correct some of those lingering brainwave imbalances that she struggled with for far too long. Trauma experts tell me that even a small trigger (forgetting to set the silverware at dinner, misplacing car keys) can potentially throw a trauma victim into full panic mode.

After over 40 sessions of Neurofeedback, I can sincerely report that Gaffney now has the life she always wanted. She creates wonderfully compelling abstract paintings, plays guitar, and makes friends wherever she goes. I have witnessed her transformation first hand because she also heads my Neurofeedback Division. She is a kind and trusted friend and a tender and sweet spirit. Everyone who knows Gaffney has been touched in some way by her zeal for life and compassion for others. I'm just so glad that I was able to play a small role in breaking that butterfly from her lifelong cocoon of trauma.

KEVIL: TESTICULAR CANCER

My son Kevil was diagnosed with stage-four testicular cancer in 2006. His diagnosis was utterly devastating. The first Oncologist recommended making an incision from sternum to groin to extract the tumors then undergo 15 consecutive weeks of chemotherapy and radiation. We sought a second opinion who similarly recommended the same course of treatment in a different order. He recommended 15 weeks of chemotherapy and radiation first, followed by the removal of tumors, followed by more chemotherapy and radiation.

After much soul-searching and deep contemplation my son made a decision to forgo traditional cancer care. He explained that he was visited by an angel in the middle of the night who assured him there was nothing to worry about and all would be fine. I remember the night of Kevil's divine visitation clearly. He came to my room and woke me moments after his experience. I sensed his peace and felt that whatever he had just experienced must have been positive and true.

But my feelings were mixed. I was glad that my son's heart was at ease but also feared that "doing nothing" would place him at risk. I spent every spare moment researching non-traditional options. As a result I started Kevil on a Vitamin C with Glutathione IV regimen.

After weeks of this therapy I urged my son to ask for a follow-up CT scan. To our surprise, the follow-up CT scan revealed no tumors and his blood tests indicated that he was cancer-free.

I anticipated a phone call from the oncologist congratulating me on the interventions I had used that resulted in Kevil's clean bill of health. I did receive a phone call; however, an invalidating one. The oncologist disregarded the results stating that "it doesn't matter what the follow-up test revealed." "My son would be dead within six months," he warned, if he did not receive chemotherapy. He stood firm. The doctor added that if my son had been under the age of 18 that he would actually have me arrested for reckless endangerment of a minor. He assured me that Kevil would die and that I would then have to consider myself a murderer.

As a parent, I wondered every night if supporting Kevil's decision was the right decision. As a doctor, quite honestly treating cancer was new territory. After exhaustive research I learned that Gerson Therapy had the highest success rate. Regardless of the outcome, I was and am still humbled by my son's commitment to his own internal voice and unwavering guiding principles.

Gerson Therapy also provided a Cancer "Thriver's" support program that paired Kevil with a cancer survivor who offered support, guidance and compassion. My son benefited greatly from this relationship. Having someone who "has been there" provided great comfort and normalized his experience.

Kevil, a disciplined and focused force of nature, followed the Gerson Protocol in Bristol fashion. Eleven years later Kevil is now a Cancer Thriver himself. He selflessly offers the same support that was given so freely to him. Kevil has participated in three Triathlons, and one-half IRONMAN®. He bravely shared his story in Ty Bollinger's The Truth about Cancer and was featured in the informational video regarding Gerson Therapy which can be found on The Gerson Therapy Institute's website.

Recent statistics report that one out of two people will be diagnosed with some form of cancer. Kevil's cancer diagnosis was not a death sentence. It was; however, certainly a strong siren indicating that his body and health was severely out of balance. I've always felt in my core that committing to keeping your body in a state of balance, physically, emotionally, chemically and spiritually your body will heal itself. New information has even further impacted this overall view.

Dr. Bruce Lipton is an American developmental biologist best known for promoting the idea that genes and DNA are influenced by a person's thoughts, emotions, diet, and other key 'environmental' factors. His work goes against the established scientific view that genes control life, which has meant he has met with strong resistance by many of his peers. Dr. Lipton has championed 'new biology' among the general public. He is the author of the bestselling book, *The Biology of Belief*, and is a former researcher at Stanford University's School of Medicine.

Dr. Lipton's unending research has influenced my life and practice on all levels. I highly recommend his books to anyone who desires to understand the human experience.

DR KATE: ASTHMA

I SUFFERED FROM asthma from an early age. Multiple doctors attributed the cause of my sneezing, wheezing, and chronic red eyes to dog, dust, and other environmental allergens.

During certain seasons there were brief periods that I was not affected. When I relocated to the Carolinas; however, my symptoms worsened. Every October I would be stricken with pneumonia or another acute respiratory illness and be resigned to use an inhaler. My symptoms were so severe that they prohibited me to be present and attuned to my patients. Truth be told, the quality of my life and practice suffered.

As a doctor I did my best to be attuned to and to treat my own symptoms. That approach; however, wasn't working.

As part of my ongoing training and personal curiosity I attended a King Bio seminar and listened to Paul Barritaro's detailed explanation of the benefits of his Echo Water Purifier system. I owned a water purification system at the time so I took advantage of the opportunity to raise my hand and ask "So Paul really, level with me here, everyone says they have the best of the best, why is your water purification system so different?"

At that moment Paul invited me to drink a glass of his Echo Purified water. I gulped 4 ounces from a small paper cup. I immediately felt my chest expand and my breathing simultaneously became effortless. I requested another 4 ounces. I drank it. The second serving stirred my whole system. I excused myself from the seminar and exited quickly to the ladies' bathroom. I experienced a "very productive" bowel movement (no real way to put that delicately).

I was stunned by my body's wonderful response to the water from the Echo Water Purifier system. Needless to say (and at the risk of sounding like a product plug) I whipped out my credit card and purchased the Echo Water Purifier on the spot.

Three years have passed and I continue to drink water from the Echo Water Purifier system. My breathing has remained unencumbered since that first swallow. I also have had no need for an inhaler.

I have even adopted an outdoor cat. Though my allergic reactions from pet dander return from time to time my symptoms are not nearly as extreme. When I feel the onset of allergy-related discomfort, I simply drink 8 to 12 ounces of Echo purified water and my breathing is fully restored so I can go back to what I do best, treating patients.

CONCLUSION

I hope you find these stories informative and inspiring. It is important to know that every human being is unique. There is no "one fixes all" solution when healing chronic illnesses. The answer remains in finding the cause of dis-ease versus treating symptoms. Our present day healthcare system treats chronic health problems with crisis care and it is obvious we as a society are failing. Obesity, cancer, diabetes, autism and many chronic diseases are at a record high.

May we all be like the hummingbird, instead of running from the fire, make conscious decisions about our own bodies, hence, become our own doctors.

If you have any questions about technologies, techniques, and systems discussed in my book, or if you are interested in my future seminars please visit my website www.drkatekeville.com

I will be teaching Dr Kate Cares seminars to parents, caregivers and anyone interested in Holistic Healthcare. I will also be teaching Health Care Practioner Seminars.

THE BENEFITS OF ECHO HYDROGEN ENRICHED WATER

Hydrogen is #1 on the periodic table because it is tiny. Being tiny has benefits.

Hydrogen can get into any area of the body needed including membranes, joints, brain, gut, organs, lungs, eyes, ears, etc. Molecular or diatomic hydrogen is 2 atoms of hydrogen bound together. It is also referred to as H2.

In the Echo® Hydrogen Enriched Water SystemTM, H2 gas is dissolved in water. The water is the delivery system for the H2 gas which has so many benefits. The process will be explained in depth later. The molecular hydrogen (H2) gas is the reason water electrolysis was discovered in 1800. H2 is considered a strategic antioxidant because it only reacts with the most cytotoxic (cell damaging) free radicals in the cells of the body including the Hydroxyl Radical (HO*) and Superoxide. H2 has so many therapeutic benefits with every organ in the body and over 170 human disease models. Our bodies are designed to create hydrogen gas in the gut through the fermentation and digestion process. The problem is that many people have gut issues because the gut is compromised and the typical diet does not have a lot of beneficial or water soluble fiber to be broken down into hydrogen gas.

Some Benefits of Molecular Hydrogen:

- Reduces oxidative stress and Inflammation.
- Regulates over 200 Biomolecules in the body.
- Stimulates gastric ghrelin secretions. Can regulate Leptin.
- Stimulation of anaerobic microflora in the intestinal tract.
- H2 has been shown to help with Rheumatoid Arthritis and joint issues.
- 700 studies showing therapeutic effects with 170 human disease models.

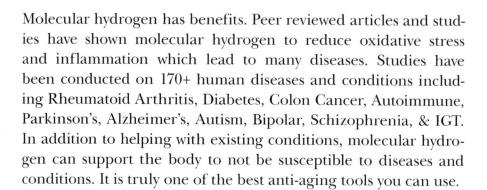

Molecular hydrogen has benefits. Peer reviewed articles and studies have shown molecular hydrogen to reduce oxidative stress and inflammation which lead to many diseases. Studies have been conducted on 170+ human diseases and conditions including Rheumatoid Arthritis, Diabetes, Colon Cancer, Autoimmune, Parkinson's, Alzheimer's, Autism, Bipolar, Schizophrenia, & IGT. In addition to helping with existing conditions, molecular hydrogen can support the body to not be susceptible to diseases and conditions. It is truly one of the best anti-aging tools you can use.

I. ELECTROLYSIS: A HYDROGEN GENERATOR

In 1800, Anthony Carlisle, a surgeon in London, discovered water electrolysis. Dr. Carlisle discovered electrolysis because he wanted to make a hydrogen generator. Dr. Carlisle wanted a way to produce hydrogen gas easily because he learned in 1798 that hydrogen had antioxidant properties. Traditional electrolysis converts water (H_2O) to hydrogen gas (H_2) and hydroxide ions ($OH-$) at the negative side (cathode), and oxygen gas (O_2) and hydrogen ions ($H+$) at the positive side (anode). Traditional water electrolysis machines have standard membranes that separates the alkaline OH ions from the acidic H+ions if you are separating the water streams. Another method of electrolysis is designed to only produce H_2 in neutral (7pH) water. In this method, the water is not separated into alkaline and acid streams. Proton Exchange Membranes (PEM) are used instead of standard membranes. The advantage of the PEM is that it creates its own conductivity in water and can produce H_2 gas even in pure water with no minerals. We must remember that the benefits do not come from the pH of the water. The pH change is simply a by process of electrolysis. It is the H_2 gas dissolved in the water that provides the therapeutic benefits. All other standard electrolysis systems that create alkaline water are not effectively able to dissolve H_2 gas in the water longer than a few weeks because of design flaws and natural law. Positively charged minerals naturally want to bond to the negatively charged cathode (see graphic above). If minerals build up on the cathode, H2 gas will not be in the water because the hydrogen bubbles will be too large to be dissolved. The H2 gas will go out and the benefits with it. In the Echo® 9 Ultra H2 system, the patented technology changes the charge of the electrodes every time the machine is used which is the only way to make it impossible for minerals to build up. This guarantees H2 gas will always be dissolved in the water. With other electrolysis systems, minerals will build up within 2-3 weeks of use and the benefits will be gone. The other companies tell consumers that they have automatic reverse cleaning systems in their machines to be confusing. They say that their systems change the polarity of the electrodes to further deceive but they don't do this every time the machine is used. They only change the polarity every 10L or 20L of water and by then the minerals are already bonded and the damage is done. With these inferior systems, the only way to keep the minerals off the cathode is to clean the system every 2 weeks with citric acid or commercial vinegar. Of course, you don't have to worry about this with any of the Echo® branded systems because it impossible for the minerals to bond to the cathode in the first place.

II. BENEFITS OF ECHO® WATER

Everyone is talking about how free radicals are damaging our cells. What most people don't know is that many free radicals are beneficial to health. It is only the cell damaging (cytotoxic) radicals that we need to scavenge. H2 converts these cells damaging hydroxyl radicals) into water molecules. Once the oxidative burden is reduced in the cells of the body, the body can naturally produce glutathione.

ATHLETIC PERFORMANCE:

Enriched WaterTM has helped many athletes increase performance. It better empowers you to function at optimal efficiency by ridding the cells of Hydroxyl Radicals allowing the mitochondria to produce energy more efficiently. It helps to reduce fatigue to help you perform longer because H2 lessens lactate in muscles. Recovery times can be cut in half. When a person is properly hydrated with Echo® hydrogen-enriched water, they perform at peak levels longer.

DETOXIFICATION AND WEIGHT LOSS:

Echo® water supports healthy cleansing and weight loss. When the toxins and waste is flushed, the burden on the body is lessened. Echo® Water can help to clean out the intestines and colon. People report that they feel more hydrated, have more success with their weight loss programs, they experience more productive sleep, wake up more alert, have fewer allergy symptoms, and feel more energy throughout the day. H2 stimulates gastric Ghrelin and Leptin. These are master hormones in the body that regulate fat storing.

IMMUNE BOOST:

No one enjoys getting sick because life comes to a screeching halt. The immune system and the digestive system are directly linked to hydration. Being properly hydrated is one of the best steps to increase your immune system and preventing sickness and disease. Remember, 60-75% of your body is water and it should be no surprise that the type of water you drink can directly influences the way you feel. Hydrogen Enriched WaterTM can help clean out the intestinal tract. The health of your gut is directly related to your susceptibility to disease and sickness. H2 can help repair gut issues by stimulating anaerobic microflora in the intestinal tract. This can help keep the intestinal tract healthier and your immune system to be less susceptible.

INTRINSIC ENERGY AND FREQUENCIES:

Many people understand that energy and frequencies are all around us. Radio frequencies, cell phone frequencies, Infrared energies, EMF's, etc. There are good and bad energies and frequencies. Some individuals use energies to benefit individuals in need. The Echo® system has hundreds of beneficial energies and frequencies that can protect you from harmful frequencies and energies. They also balance chakras and help the body heal. Those that are intuitive can feel them immediately. Others say that the water just feels good to them. Professionals in energy medicine, Cranial Sacral Therapists, Reiki Masters, etc. love and recommend Echo® water because of these beneficial energies and frequencies.

PROPER HYDRATION:

Because Echo® water tastes so great, you will be drinking more water. A study conducted by the University of Utah, showed the more water you drink the better. In the study, subjects consumed either 4, 8 or 12 glasses of water daily. On the fifth day before rising, their hydration status was monitored and a computer measured how many calories they had burned in a resting state. The groups who drank 8 and 12 glasses of water daily were sufficiently hydrated, whereas subjects who drank only four showed definite signs of dehydration. The well-hydrated subjects reported better concentration and more energy. They burned more calories at rest than the group who drank only 4 glasses. These results were in line with the previous 3 University of Utah findings that the ability to burn calories can decline by about 2% per day when people are dehydrated. Metabolic rate and digestion is increased by being properly hydrated. Increased Cognitive Function - Ghrelin: Help with Neurological Conditions Studies show that H2 stimulates Ghrelin secretions. Ghrelin is known as the hunger hormone in the body. Ghrelin affects many things in the body including cognitive function, hunger, weight regulation, anti-inflammatory

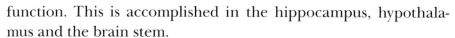

function. This is accomplished in the hippocampus, hypothalamus and the brain stem.

Specific studies have shown that water with H2 dissolved can be helpful with neurologic pathology like Parkinson's, Alzheimer's, Bipolar, Schizophrenia, and Autism.

III. STUDY REFERENCES:

1. www.synergyscience.com/studies
2. www.synergyscience.com/studies
3. http://healthcare.utah.edu/publicaffairs/news/archive/2003/news_74.php

DISCLAIMER:

There are hundreds of studies showing molecular hydrogen to have therapeutic benefits. Please visit www.synergyscience.com/studies to read additional clinical studies. They are continually being added.

The below studies are shared for educational purposes only. They are not shared to indicate any outcome for anyone with a similar or same disease or pathology. The results achieved in the studies should not be taken as an indicator of results you will accomplish. The study shows potential outcomes. There are no protocols, drugs, natural methods, or techniques that are 100% effective. Every individual is different and diseases are complex.

ALTERNATIVE TECHNIQUES AND SYSTEMS

Holographic Health. Holographic Health is a comprehensive method of determining one's overall health picture and framing it in the system both the client and practitioner can understand. Extensive testing is done to help the practitioner know exactly what the client needs. Next an individualized thorough program of bodywork and nutritional supplementation is employed to assist the client and return to better health.

Applied Kinesiology. Applied Kinesiology (AK) is the study of body movement. AK is a method of diagnosis and treatment based on the theory that certain muscles are directly linked to particular organs and glands. Furthermore, that specific muscle weakness can insinuate distant internal problems such as nerve damage, reduced blood supply, chemical imbalances or other internal problems. Practitioners contend that by correcting muscle weakness consequently remedies problems with the associated internal organ.

Bioenergetics. Bioenergetics is based on the belief that there is a correlation between the mind and the body. The therapy combines work with the body and mind to help people resolve their emotional problems and realize more of their potential for pleasure and joy in living.

Gerson Therapy. Gerson Therapy is a natural treatment that activates the body's innate ability to heal itself through an organic, plant-based diet, raw juices, coffee enemas and natural supplements. The treatment has been found to be effective in enhancing the immune system and treating symptoms of a wide range of diseases and conditions.

Medi Cupping. Medi Cupping or "Cupping" is a traditional treatment that used suction rather than compression for bodywork. Cupping expedites soft tissue release and enables water absorption and renewed blood and lymph flow to undernourished tissues. This restorative process rehabilitates skin and muscles in ways not possible with traditional massage techniques.

Myofascial Release. The John F. Barnes' Myofascial Release Approach® is considered to be the ultimate therapy that is safe, gentle and consistently effective in producing results that last. John F. Barnes, PT has trained over 100,000 therapists and physicians, is an international lecturer, author and authority on Myofascial Release. He is a physical therapist and is considered to be a visionary and teacher of the highest caliber.

Trauma, inflammatory responses, and/or surgical procedures create Myofascial restrictions that can produce tensile pressures of approximately 2,000 pounds per square inch on pain sensitive structures that do not show up in many of the standard tests (x-rays, myelograms, CAT scans, electromyography, etc.)

The medical approach is to drug patients so they temporarily are free from pain, but does nothing about the "straightjacket" of pressure that is causing the pain. Traditional physical, occupational and massage therapy treats the symptoms caused by the pressure of the "straightjacket" of the Myofascial system, but does nothing about the "straightjacket" of pressure that causes and perpetuates the symptoms. This is why so many patients only have temporary results never seeming to get better with traditional therapy. Myofascial Release treats the entire Myofascial mind/body complex eliminating the pressure of the restricted Myofascial system (the straightjacket) that causes the symptoms.

Neural Integration System. Neural Integration System (NIS) What is NIS about?

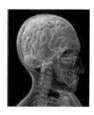

Your brain is a powerful piece of machinery. At the center of your nervous system your brain controls all conscious actions, like your thoughts, feelings and memories. And it controls all automatic actions like your heartbeat, blood pressure, body temperature and breathing.

The NIS system bases its treatment method on the scientific principle that the brain governs 'optimum function' of all the body's systems.

As long as the **neurology (brain)** is communicating appropriately with the **physiology (body),** we should be operating at 'optimum function'.

As we go about our daily lives we are exposed to different types of stresses. Stresses can be Physical, Pathological, Neurological or Emotional. For the most part our bodies are designed to handle these. **Example 1**

But from time to time these stresses can push you past your usual 'tolerance' level – causing the signal between brain and body to become disconnected.

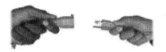

And because the signal is not getting through, your brain no longer has complete control of that particular area of your physiology (body).

When an area of physiology is no longer under the control of the brain, it will stop functioning to its optimum and you then begin to experience symptom/s. (There are over 600,000 possible symptoms that the body is capable of!)

Symptoms are your body's way of saying that things are not working as they should be or to 'optimum function'. **Example 2**

The NIS system uses latest scientific research to 'tap' into the intelligence of your brain to identify which signals are not

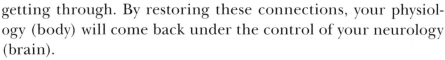

getting through. By restoring these connections, your physiology (body) will come back under the control of your neurology (brain).

Neuro Emotional Technique. Neuro Emotional Technique (NET) is a breakthrough mind-body technique that helps find and remove neurological imbalances stored in our bodies as unresolved stress. Emotions such as fear, anger, grief and many others can negatively affect us long after the original event that caused them. NET provides a way for our body to release fear, anger, grief and other negative emotions so that our body's homeostasis is restored.

Neurofeedback. Neurofeedback (NFB) also called neurotherapy or neurobiofeedback. Neurofeedback is a type of biofeedback that uses real time displays of brain activity most commonly electroencephalography (EEG) to teach self-regulation of brain function. Biofeedback has been employed as a non-invasive treatment for depression, anxiety, autism, addiction, epilepsy, pain, anxiety, Tourette syndrome, children with ADHD, and many other conditions.

Reflexology. Reflexology is the application of appropriate pressure to specific points and areas on the feet, hands, or ears. Reflexologists believe that these reflex points correspond to different body organs and systems, and that pressing them has a beneficial effect on the person's health.

CranioSacral Therapy (CST) was pioneered and developed by osteopathic physician **John E. Upledger** following extensive scientific studies from 1975 to 1983 at Michigan State University, where he served as a clinical researcher and Professor of Biomechanics.

CST is a gentle, hands-on method of evaluating and enhancing the functioning of a physiological body system called the craniosacral system - comprised of the membranes and cerebrospinal fluid that surround and protect the brain and spinal cord.

Using a soft touch generally no greater than 5 grams, or about the weight of a nickel, practitioners release restrictions in the craniosacral system to improve the functioning of the central nervous system.

By complementing the body's natural healing processes, CST is increasingly used as a preventive health measure for its ability to bolster resistance to disease, and is effective for a wide range of medical problems associated with pain and dysfunction, including:

- Migraine Headaches
- Chronic Neck and Back Pain
- Motor-Coordination Impairments
- Colic
- Autism
- Central Nervous System Disorders
- Orthopedic Problems
- Concussions and Traumatic Brain Injuries
- Alzheimer's Disease and Dementia
- Spinal Cord Injuries
- Scoliosis
- Infantile Disorders
- Learning Disabilities
- Chronic Fatigue
- Emotional Difficulties
- Stress and Tension-Related Problems
- Fibromyalgia and other Connective-Tissue Disorders
- Temporomandibular Joint Syndrome (TMJ)
- Neurovascular or Immune Disorders
- Post-Traumatic Stress Disorder
- Post-Surgical Dysfunction

SomatoEmotional Release (SER) is a therapeutic process that uses and expands on the principles of CranioSacral Therapy to help rid the mind and body of the residual effects of trauma. SER1 offers applications designed to enhance results using CST and other complementary therapies.

- Assess and mobilize the Avenue of Expression working through more than 10 different body components, including the thoracic inlet, hard palate and hypoglossal tissues.
- Locate and release Energy Cysts.
- Release suppressed emotions that may be inhibiting complete structural releases.
- Refine listening and comprehension skills.
- Improve palpation and whole-body evaluation skills.

ABOUT THE AUTHOR

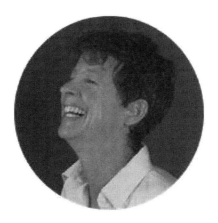

Dr. Kate Keville was born and raised in Bellevue, Ohio. She received a bachelor's degree in education from Ohio State University and a doctorate of chiropractic from Sherman College. She has spent years helping patients relieve their pain and achieve healthier lives through holistic treatments. Her son, Kevil Murray, was diagnosed with terminal cancer. Dr. Keville supported him and watched as he miraculously healed himself.

Before becoming a health care professional, Dr. Keville worked in military intelligence for the US Army and owned and operated four vegetarian restaurants. She is a public speaker, has appeared on several radio shows, has run five marathons, several triathlons, and half an Ironman race. Dr. Keville teaches seminars nationwide.

Please visit her website www.drkatekeville.com

The techniques, methods, and systems discussed in this book are intended to support health and healing. NOT to replace medical treatment. It should not be interpreted as medical advice, and is not intended to treat, diagnose, or cure your condition, or to be a substitute for your advice from your physician or health care professional. Whether you choose convential treatments, alternative treatments, or both, it is imperative that you work closely with a healthcare professional to properly diagnose and treat your condition, and to monitor your progress.

Made in the USA
Columbia, SC
15 October 2017